Caring for a Loved One with AIDS
The Experiences of Families, Lovers, and Friends

Marie Annette Brown
Gail M. Powell-Cope

Published for
the University of Washington School of Nursing
by
the University of Washington Press
Seattle and London

Acknowledgments

We would like to thank Laura K. Utterback for rewriting our academic papers on AIDS caregivers into booklet form. Her creativity brought this project to life, and her insight and heartfelt concern about this topic inspired us.

We appreciate the initial financial support to conduct our research project on which we based this booklet. Thank you to Sigma Theta Tau, Psi Chapter, and the Biomedical Research Support Grant Program at the University of Washington School of Nursing.

Thanks also to the kind souls who read our first or final draft and encouraged us onward or provided substantive and helpful feedback: Phil Boreano, Susan Joslyn, Irene Peters, Barbara Schlieper, Sondra Lee, Mary Ann Gonzales, and Graham Shutt.

Thanks to the University of Washington School of Nursing Office of Community Relations, and to Susanna Cunningham for seeing the potential in our work and helping us through the system. Thanks to Pat Simpson, graphic designer, for her talent and knowledge.

In addition to "family caregivers," there are numerous other people such as community volunteers, other family, friends, co-workers, and professionals who provide help and emotional support. These AIDS caregivers can make a huge difference in the quality of life for both the ill person and the family caregiver. While the experiences described in this booklet are about the AIDS family caregiver, other AIDS caregivers may find they can relate to these stories of taking care of someone with AIDS.

How To Use This Book

Keep this booklet on hand. Even though it isn't a "how to" book about AIDS caregiving, it might make you feel a little less frustrated when caregiving gets rough.

You see, you're not alone. Thousands of people across the country are AIDS family caregivers. The experiences we describe in this booklet came from people from all walks of life who had been caregiving anywhere from a few months to a few years.

As you read their stories, think about the similarities or differences between their situations and yours. And, while you will notice some resemblance between the experiences of AIDS caregivers, remember that no two situations are alike.

What will apply to every situation is uncertainty—a fundamental part of AIDS family caregiving. Uncertainty is always there, though its intensity varies from time to time. The knowledge that there is no "correct" way to be a caregiver may reduce the stress caregivers place on themselves. We hope to help caregivers identify, expect, and accept uncertainty as part of the caregiving experience.

Also, we hope to point out that for most people caregiving is a life-changing event. The process of caregiving provides many challenges, some painful and difficult, others full of satisfaction and peace. Being an AIDS family caregiver permanently alters the way you look at the world. Your life will not be the same after this experience.

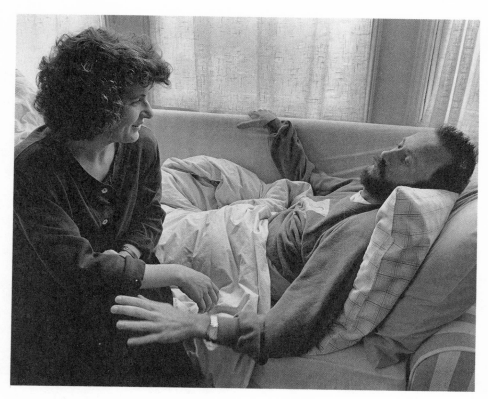

"I don't necessarily feel one hundred percent
about everything I'm doing, but I have to do it.
I'm not one hundred percent positive, one
hundred percent sure that it's the right thing
to do for him. It becomes very obscure, blurry,
as to whether I'm doing anything right."

What Is an AIDS Family Caregiver?

Lovers, family members, and friends assume heavy responsibilities for the care of a person with AIDS. It's often the family caregiver, the person in charge of the sick person's care, who makes the biggest difference in the sick person's overall well-being. The family caregiver oversees the sick person's household, takes the sick person to the doctor, helps with medicines and injections, and performs countless other tasks. Without these important day-to-day caregiving activities, there would be large gaps in the sick person's care, more persons with AIDS placed in institutions, and a greater need for paid professional caregiving. Reliance on one or more family caregivers is usually the only way for a person with AIDS to remain at home, especially the very ill or mentally impaired person who has trouble with the tasks of everyday life.

Family caregivers don't have to be blood relatives. "Family" can mean biological family members, such as parents, brothers, and sisters. Or, it can mean family members you choose, such as lovers, spouses, and friends. What matters is that the caregiver is someone who feels a connection to the person with AIDS, and cares enough to commit to the caregiving role.

AIDS FAMILY CAREGIVERS

LOVER

PARENT   HUSBAND

BROTHER (PERSON WITH AIDS) WIFE

SISTER   AUNT

CLOSE FRIEND

Even though family caregivers play a pivotal role in AIDS care, little is known about their experiences. Although studies have been done with families providing care for other groups of ill persons, such as cancer patients and the elderly, literature on the specific problems of family members of persons with AIDS is difficult to find. This booklet is written from a University of Washington School of Nursing study we conducted to find out more about the experiences and special needs of AIDS family caregivers.

Caring For a Loved One With AIDS is for people who are caregivers, people who are about to start caregiving, and people who just want to find out more about the experiences of a family caregiver. It is not so much a "self-help" book as a description of what these caregivers experienced, complete with excerpts taken from interviews with the caregivers.

BECOMING AN AIDS FAMILY CAREGIVER

Many people don't recall consciously choosing to take on the caregiver role. Instead, they just assumed they were the logical choice, given the nature of their relationship to the person with AIDS. The parent of a young child with AIDS, a longtime lover of a person with AIDS, the best friend of a person with AIDS, or someone else with a strong emotional connection to the sick person may feel that his or her choice is already made, and he or she becomes the primary caregiver without a second thought. For others, however, motives to begin and continue caregiving vary. Most commonly, caregivers care deeply about the person with AIDS, and want to help them. For lovers and biological family members in particular, becoming a caregiver is a way to honor a commitment, live one's spiritual or philosophical values, or fulfill a sense of duty and obligation. For some, a commitment to the "community" can be a sufficient incentive, whether that is defined as the gay or lesbian community or humanity as a whole.

TALKING WITH CAREGIVERS

The caregivers who participated in our study came from all walks of life: salespersons, truck drivers, musicians, university professors, homemakers, students. They responded to a flyer about the study distributed throughout the Seattle area, or heard about the study from a friend. Over fifty family caregivers of persons with AIDS agreed to be interviewed. We spoke to each caregiver individually. In the interviews, we asked, "What has it been like for you living with and taking care of someone with AIDS?" The sessions, which lasted from two to six hours each, were tape recorded and transcribed.

WHAT WE FOUND:
THE FIVE ASPECTS OF CAREGIVING

As we reviewed the caregivers' stories, we discovered that many caregivers shared common experiences and concerns. From these common links, we developed five main aspects of AIDS caregiving. These five categories are the ones we discuss individually in the chapters of this booklet.

FIVE ASPECTS OF AIDS CAREGIVING

1. Living With Loss and Dying, revising one's plans based on the possible or probable death of a loved one;

2. Managing and Being Managed By the Illness, monitoring the unpredictable illness of AIDS and responding to the relentless demands associated with caregiving;

3. Renegotiating the Relationship, constantly revising the rules and expectations of the relationship between the caregiver and the person with AIDS;

4. Going Public, the experience of concealing or revealing one's association with AIDS or HIV infection;

5. Containing the Spread of HIV, the strategies used to prevent transmission of the disease to the caregiver and others.

Besides these five categories, we also identified two general experiences common to many of the caregivers.

GENERAL EXPERIENCES COMMON TO CAREGIVERS

*   The uncertainty a caregiver faces in all aspects of this disease.
*   The idea that caregiving is a process which brings about a change in the caregiver's life.

These two experiences have an incredible impact on the lives of caregivers. In the next section, we discuss the uncertainty caregivers feel when dealing with the disease, and the profound changes that many feel in their lives during and after caregiving.

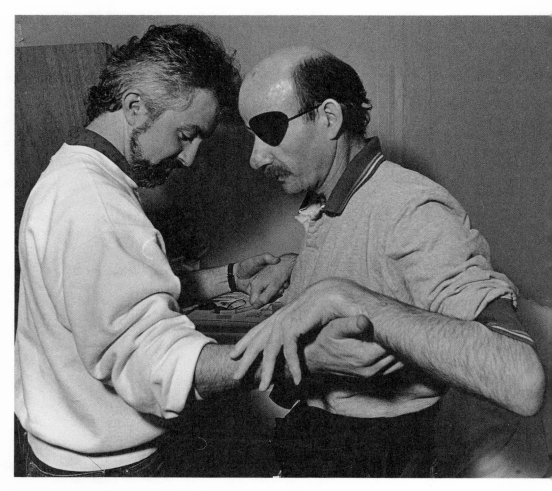

"The roller coaster describes the situation in lots of different ways. What's happening to the person's health? What's happening to your feelings? What's happened here today? It's this incredible uncertainty."

Dealing With Uncertainty and the Process of Caregiving

The caregivers we spoke to described uncertainty, the inability to predict what would happen next with the disease, as one of the greatest difficulties of caregiving. Constant change accompanies AIDS, and the sick person's health and abilities can shift dramatically over a few hours. Even doctors, nurses, and people who have been caregiving for years are unable to predict precisely what will happen with the disease from day to day, and nobody is ever entirely sure that a certain care decision is the correct one.

Yet, in our culture, with its emphasis on science and logical thought, we want to understand and control events. Since we have so much information about AIDS, why can't we foresee what's going to happen next? Unlike people who care for patients of other diseases, AIDS caregivers find they have to plan for uncertainty rather than for particular stages of the disease. This feeling is uncomfortable for people used to exactness, especially in the realm of medicine.

One caregiver, a businessman accustomed to precision and organization in his work, felt frustrated when doctors couldn't explain his partner's new neurological symptoms:

He's got a malfunction in his brain, and no one knows what's going on. The neurosurgeons and neurologists and doctors at the AIDS clinic—no one knows what's happening, but it's getting worse.

Asked to describe the emotional impact of the frequently violent unpredictability of AIDS, many caregivers found a fitting metaphor for the constant ups and downs and lack of control:

The roller coaster describes the situation in lots of different ways. What's happening to the person's health? What's happening to your feelings? What's happened here today? It's this incredible uncertainty.

Caregivers also feel uncertain about the day-to-day decisions they make for the care of the person with AIDS. What should they look for? How do they know when a seemingly innocent symptom means something else? Even after a year of caregiving, one lover confessed self-doubt:

I don't necessarily feel one hundred per-cent about everything I'm doing, but I have to do it. I'm not one hundred per-cent positive, one hundred percent sure, that it's the right thing to do for Mike. It becomes very obscure, blurry, as to whether I'm doing anything right.

This uncertainty also focuses on choices of new treatments and drugs which have a short history of testing. Caregivers are concerned about whether they can obtain and afford new drugs, what the short- and long-term effects are if the drugs work, or whether to encourage alternative thera-pies.

And, through it all, caregivers have to grapple with the uncertainty of each new piece of information. If it's good news, is it worth getting your hopes up? If it's bad news, how will it affect what you're doing for the person with AIDS? After wavering once between hope for a cure and accepting that his lover of nine years was dying, one man eventually decided to bring an element of certainty into his situation:

I couldn't deal with the day-to-day un-certainty, and I hated hearing people say-ing to me, "There's going to be a cure." You know, 99% of the people, when you tell them that Mark has AIDS, is going to say to you, "Oh, well, they're doing wonderful things now." They try to con-

sole you. I got a little tired of that. That brought the uncertainty back into it. Well, when is this cure going to hap-pen? Is it going to happen? So I finally said, "Well, Mark is going to die," and then I was able to get on.

THE PROCESS OF CAREGIVING

If someone asked you to tell the story of your life up until now, chances are that most of the events you'd touch on would be the ones that changed the path of your life in some way—gradu-ating from school, falling in love, chang-ing careers, losing a close friend or fam-ily member. These are important events because they signal us that a new stage in life is about to start, and that we aren't quite the same person once that new stage begins. We may or may not notice it, but what we experience dur-ing these transitional times adds to our personalities, and we grow and change according to what we've learned.

Most of the caregivers we spoke to felt this way about their caregiving work. They saw caregiving as a transi-tion, a life phase that involves major change, instead of just a group of tasks they must perform. Some described caregiving as a series of changes, a jour-ney or passage, or a path they chose. The journey, which could take a few months or several years, began with the diagnosis of AIDS and ended with the sick person's death. Sometimes it extended into the months after the death.

Many caregivers reported that during the period of caregiving they learned to live their lives and view the world differently, as they sought to make meaning of caregiving events and experiences. Some said the close association with death made them appreciate life, and they vowed to live their lives more fully in the future.

Part of living life differently involved learning to appreciate themselves for the new skills they had learned and the strength they had found. The work they did was emotionally and physically difficult, and some expressed satisfaction and self-respect, proud to know they could handle such a huge responsibility. One lover realized that his experiences had given him a new sense of well-being:

It sounds hard to believe after all these things I've been telling you, but I'm very happy with the way my life is going right now. I have the most wonderful balance in the world, of working at the bakery part-time and being able to live a very bohemian life-style, working in my garden, spending what time I can with Jeff. I am at definitely the most content place in my life than I've been in many, many, many years. I don't think I would do anything different right now.

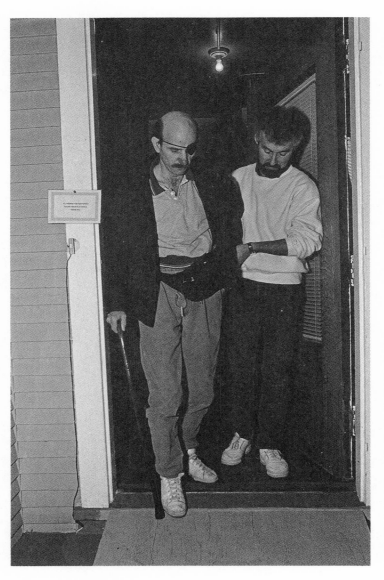

"We're proud of the fact that we've been together as long as we have—through sickness and health and all the other things said at a marriage ceremony. When a person becomes ill, do you just turn your back and walk away? I have to stay true to him, no matter how difficult it might be."

The Five Aspects of AIDS Caregiving

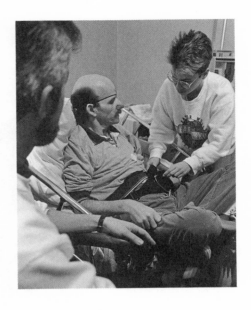

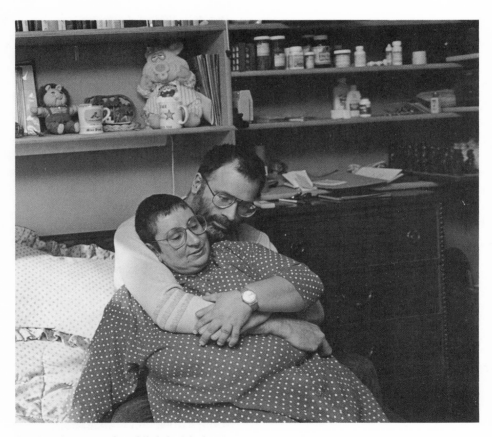

"He has shown me a lot while he's sick about
what life is all about—enjoy what you got
while you are here."

Living With Loss and Dying

The possible death of someone he or she cares for is the most painful loss that a caregiver faces. However, a caregiver also loses other things, such as a way of life.

As the illness progresses and changes the person with AIDS, a caregiver gradually loses the relationship with that person as he or she knew it before the illness began. The sick person's increasing limitations and loss of strength make him or her likely to withdraw from all relationships, even the closest ones. Caregivers grieve the loss of the "pre-AIDS relationship" and of emotional support from the person with AIDS. As one woman noted:

> It's the loss of our relationship. Of the person I love and his presence to me. It's not an interactive relationship any more. He responds to me, or to changes, in a way that's different. I haven't really figured it out. He's been someone important to me, and it's been a relationship where I have gotten some amount of recognition and I've been heard by him. And I don't have that important relationship any more. I'm losing a person that's an important support in my life.

This chapter deals with the difficult task of coping with the different types of losses you'll face during caregiving.

LETTING GO OF THE PAST

Loss of their relationship with the sick person forces caregivers to rethink their definition of what "normal life" should be, and to let go of the lives they led prior to caregiving. The reevaluation may occur gradually; for instance, the caregiver may notice everyday events, such as recreational or social activities, become less frequent as the sick person's energy diminishes. At other times, change occurs abruptly; for example, the caregiver's round-the-clock presence may suddenly be required during an acute infection, and this harrowing experience changes forever the caregiver's perception of his or her role in the person with AIDS's life. Some caregivers easily let go of their past life-style; others experience intense emotions, particularly anger, about a life-style that has been taken away.

Letting go of the past helps caregivers accommodate the new priorities of caregiving, and allows caregivers to direct their energy toward living with current uncertainties, especially those directly associated with the health of the person with AIDS. All dimensions of the caregiver's life are affected: daily activities, goals, plans for the future, and expectations of self and others. A woman in her early thirties, caring for her hemophiliac life partner who had AIDS, spoke of their decisions about raising children:

I can't have kids so we planned to adopt together, and...I told him that I'm going to put this on hold unless something comes along that guarantees that he's going to be around for a while.

LETTING GO OF THE FUTURE

A caregiver also lets go of plans for his or her future and the future of the person with AIDS, and recognizes that many dreams, such as a couple's ideal home or a parent's aspirations for their son, will never be realized. One caregiver admitted to feeling "really badly" that his partner had AIDS, and that their shared goal had been taken away:

I have grieved for the losses we've had already. I'm particularly peeved at not being able to live overseas right now. We both gave up our dream of living there. But I also have had to give up quite a bit of money and an enormous amount of time.

As caregivers face the probability of an extended caregiving period and the sick person's death, they begin to rearrange how they think about the future. Many caregivers put long-term personal goals on hold and devote themselves to caregiving and to day-to-day living. One caregiver, the lover of the sick person, is a musician who hesitated to make plans for out-of-town performances. He explained:

A lot of long-term goals of mine have just been placed on a back burner and are just kind of waiting. Sometimes, you really wait and wonder. You wait for a cure. You wait for a new treatment. You wait for him to die. A lot of waiting, and putting a lot of things on hold while you're waiting.

Preoccupation with the responsibilities and emotional strain of caregiving leaves little energy for long-term planning. One mother talked about her sadness at giving up her plans for the traveling she longed to do when she and her husband retired. She said:

...[it's] basically what I've been concentrating on: the immediate future. There's not a whole lot of long-range planning that I've really felt comfortable doing.

Yet even the immediate future—tomorrow, this weekend—becomes contingent on the present symptoms and strength of the person with AIDS. Caregivers often find that the idea of living "one day at a time" becomes an anchor in their struggle for emotional equilibrium.

When the sick person's health is relatively good, a caregiver may take a risk and plan an activity, such as a weekend trip. At other times, he or she may cautiously plan activities in light of the ill person's limitations. However, the uncertainty of what will happen next with AIDS can defy even the most carefully arranged plans. A lover caregiver, who had been with his partner nine years, described an attempt at an outing:

Our life is definitely changed, especially most recently—going on day trips. We went to Port Townsend a couple of weeks ago. We were only there twenty minutes, and Mike wanted to go home. You know, that's a two-hour drive, so it's not just around the corner. And he wanted to go home. I didn't question why, and I took him home. Those kind of days are gone right now. We have no more of that exploration.

Repeated disappointments often lead to the caregiver's eventual acceptance that many future plans will remain unrealized: no matter how well the future is thought out, AIDS will ultimately take over. A friend of a person with AIDS, who became his lover and caregiver after the AIDS diagnosis, described this mental state:

He has AIDS. You take one day at a time most of the time. There's always a threat hanging over; there's always a little bit of tension, and so you have to be very conscious of what's going on. It's always in the back of your mind.

As the person in his or her care gets sicker, a caregiver may contemplate short-term caregiving plans—but not in great detail. Caregivers may experience a vague and uncomfortable feeling that the future could become difficult for the person with AIDS as well as for themselves. Because of this, caregivers often avoid imagining specific scenes of their future caregiving activities and the final phases of the sick person's life; many times, they decide to "cross that bridge when they come to it." A woman caring for her twenty-two-year-old son who returned to live with her after diagnosis stated:

I'm going to stick by him until the end. We're going to try to give him a home as long as we can. I think I can keep him home. I don't think I can deal with tubes and I.V.s and things like that at home, but for the most of it—we'll just worry about that when we have to. Now we're managing pretty good.

Since caregivers are faced with many unknowns—which symptoms or infections will appear, whether there will be abrupt death or lengthy deterioration, how much caregiving stress they'll be able to handle—they may give little attention to preparing themselves or the household for future caregiving demands. If they do give attention to the future, it's often in the form of anxiety or worry, particularly about the possibility of having to cope with the ill person's mental deterioration or long, slow dying process sometime in the future. A sister, who was juggling children and employment while caring for her brother, voiced her concern:

Truly, I don't know how he's going to do, and for some reason it just isn't psychologically suitable for me to focus on the impending illness and death, though I know what the statistics are. Not that it doesn't worry me. I do worry about that, and it is a burden—a psychological burden that we're never free of.

LONG-TERM PLANS

While most caregivers avoid planning for the future, some find comfort in making long-term plans. Some caregivers intend to make specific life changes such as traveling, changing jobs, selling the house, or entering school after the sick person's death. These plans may remain either relatively undeveloped, or carefully thought out and then consciously put on hold. Sometimes caregivers and persons with AIDS talk openly about the caregiver's future, and the ill person may even encourage the caregiver to develop long-term plans. Other caregivers and persons with AIDS avoid discussing the caregiver's long-term plans, because acknowledging the possibility that one of them will be gone can be uncomfortable. One caregiver, a student who works part-time at a grocery store, described his need to plan in secret:

I don't get a lot of support to think about, or plan for life after Rob, and so I pretty much do that on my own, when no one is watching. Feels kind of strange. I can understand how that may not be something Rob may want to participate in, but...everything used to be a joint decision that we wanted to make together.

The time when both the short- and

long-term future is furthest from the caregiver's mind is during acute health crises, or during the final phase of the sick person's life. When death appears imminent, the caregiver usually puts everything on hold. All other activities become secondary as the process of dying begins and the caregiver's experience is pervaded by the pain of loss. One woman recalled the terrifying feeling that her friend with AIDS was about to die:

It was, "My God, this is a very difficult moment." And being overwhelmed. You know, there's no level of anticipation or preparation when you feel that this could be "it."

During the final stages of the disease, some persons with AIDS, though conscious and able to hear, may lose the ability to speak, move, or see. Many caregivers found at this point that their mere presence, sitting by the bed and talking to the sick person, was the most important thing. Caregivers in our study described these long hours as an opportunity to lose themselves in thought. They reviewed and evaluated their caregiving experience, the sick person's life, and their relationship with this person. Parents looked back on events from a child's life, or thought about what their child might have become. Loved ones regretted having ar-

gued with the person with AIDS during the illness. At this point, the moments of "now" are sometimes too painful to think about. Instead, the caregiver remembers their past together and the good parts of life with the sick person, and feels comforted with warm memories of the past.

MAKING THE MOST OF THE PRESENT

The possibility of suddenly losing the person with AIDS often motivates caregivers to live differently in the present. The ill person's vulnerability to opportunistic, devastating infections (especially Pneumocystis pneumonia), with their threat of unexpected death, creates a sense of urgency. A priest who lives in a group home, giving care to his friend and colleague with AIDS, said:

He talked about the urgency of the things that he did, of not feeling that he had that much time. Those are powerful things to hear, and you honor them very, very much. But they're necessary to hear, too. Otherwise, it's kind of in a mist, you know; it's like, "Well, is he better? Can we go back to the old way? Can we go back to when you were good"— meaning healthy—"or can we go back to when we didn't know all this about you?" And you go, "No, you can't. This is what you have."

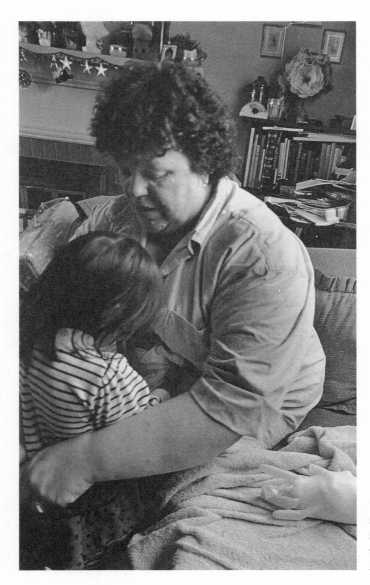

*"Do you know how hard
it is for me to realize
that my youngest child
will probably die before
I do?"*

Caregivers try to make the most of the present for themselves and persons with AIDS by helping the sick persons live their remaining life to its fullest, and by attempting to fulfill their shared dreams.

Caregivers may also create more opportunities for emotional and physical closeness to the person with AIDS, since their remaining time together can feel like a precious commodity. Our caregivers described a certain vitality or intensity to life as they intentionally spent more time with the person with AIDS. One woman who was receiving physical disability assistance herself yet taking care of a close friend with AIDS talked about the commitment she made to live life more fully in the present:

> He has shown me a lot while he's sick about what life is all about—enjoy what you got while you are here.

To balance the profound issues of life, death, and the search for meaning, caregivers seek to maintain a "normal life" as part of maximizing the present. Some caregivers attempt to take a break from the strain of AIDS with some balancing activity, such as joining a choir, signing up for a health club, or reintroducing previously enjoyed activities, such as dancing.

SPIRITUAL ISSUES

The daily focus on life and death inspired some caregivers to explore existential and spiritual questions. One young man, who worked at a bank, hadn't thought much about these issues previously. He was surprised and pleased that he and his partner with AIDS had been able to talk to each other and change their viewpoints:

> It's a strange time for us right now. It's almost a very spiritual time. We're dealing with some life and death issues and finding our own spirituality there. It's been a real path.

Existential and spiritual concerns were of particular interest to caregivers who were HIV positive, as they began to imagine or fear their own future illness and death. One caregiver took comfort in her belief in an afterlife:

> He's frightened of my dying before him, because he wouldn't know what would happen to him if I died first. And we have this role that makes this death complete. After he's dead, there won't be much time before we're together again. And I know that when I die, I will be comforted in the thought that I'll be with him again.

A CHANGED SENSE OF TIME

As the illness progresses, caregivers spend increasing amounts of time with the persons in their care, either by choice or by necessity. A caregiver's sense of time changes as his or her life becomes more and more absorbed by care duties and the emotional stress of taking care of a person with AIDS. The perception of what is important in life narrows, and life takes on an unreal feeling as caregivers stop paying attention to normal markers of how time progresses. Many caregivers note that they feel "suspended in time," as the difference between days seems to vanish; even the difference between a weekday and a weekend disappears. Looking back on a caregiving experience is often described as looking back into a blur.

Often, however, life's pressures do not permit a caregiver's single-minded focus on the person with AIDS. Deadlines at work, conflicts and crises with other significant people, and holidays all continue to make demands on the caregiver. One parent of a nine-year-old boy with AIDS talked about balancing the demands of her other four children with those of her ill son:

Life must still go on without this. But let me tell you, we managed. I don't know how, but we managed to keep that little something there to help us get through the day.

Some caregivers in the study wished the rest of the world could come to a standstill while they faced their crisis. A mother caregiver of a young adult son commented:

I would get resentful and a little envious of friends whose kids are all healthy. Nobody else was going through this but us, you know. Everybody is just going on with their lives. Why doesn't everything just stop because my son is sick? And there's nothing I can do.

Not everyone accepts death as a natural process. AIDS is the most immediate concern in the caregiver's and the sick person's lives, and they may want to talk about it with others. But disease and death are subjects that a lot of people find too uncomfortable or embarrassing to discuss, as this caregiver, the longtime lover of a person with AIDS, discovered:

I've gotten wind that sometimes people just don't want to talk about it. Monte and I have, for some reason, since he's been diagnosed, been less and less invited out places. Monte has a way of always talking about the illness, and I have a feeling that may have something to do with it—people just don't want to hear about it any more.

You can't expect to change everyone else's attitudes about AIDS and death overnight. If a caregiver can accept the reality of loss and death, however, the caregiver may find it easier to make the most of his or her own life, as well as the life of the person with AIDS.

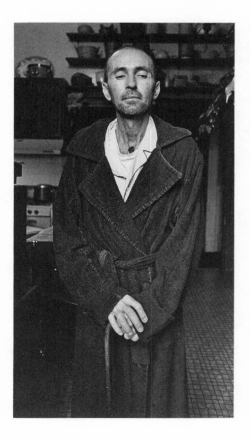

THINGS TO THINK ABOUT

- Since so many persons with AIDS eventually die, death is an inescapable part of family caregiving.

- The death of your loved one isn't the only loss you may experience. Your whole way of life may change as you lose time to yourself and your relationship with your loved one.

- It's normal to feel depressed or overwhelmed after reading this section. Sharing your feelings in a support group and listening to other caregivers' stories may help you face the losses surrounding AIDS.

- You may find that these suggestions help you cope with the many losses you'll face:
  1. Let go of how life used to be.
  2. Remember that the best-laid plans may not always work out .
  3. Live life to the fullest in the present .
  4. Take one day at a time.
  5. Explore spiritual questions or other approaches to making meaning out of life.
  6. Talk to people who aren't afraid to think about death and loss.

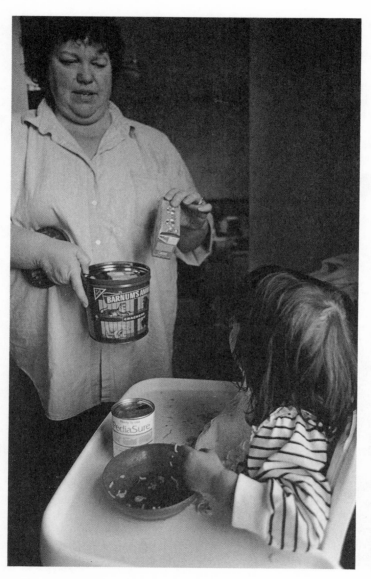

"I didn't know what caregiving was all about until I went to this caregiving class at the Red Cross, and I'm glad I went, because I learned a lot. It really helped me to understand it."

Managing and Being Managed by the Illness

The "hands-on" work of managing the illness—such as cooking and cleaning for the person with AIDS—is what most people picture when they think about family caregiving. A caregiver often becomes the sick person's housekeeper, bookkeeper, chauffeur, counselor, nurse, and social secretary all at the same time. Even if he or she is able to divide some of the jobs among other family members or volunteers, the role the primary caregiver plays has its costs. Managing the illness is the most exhausting component of family caregiving for AIDS, and coping with the extensive demands of this role usually requires considerable energy, time, and commitment. This chapter reveals a bit about care issues to expect after you've become an AIDS caregiver.

WATCHING AND ANALYZING

The family caregiver vigilantly watches and analyzes the person with AIDS in order to detect early changes in the sick person's health. Then, he or she decides if there is something that can be done to remedy the immediate situation—for example, trying a new medication, or rushing the sick person to the hospital. Even during quiet times when the sick person's health is relatively good, the caregiver is constantly alert, gathering clues and putting together facts to interpret symptoms and behavior of the person with AIDS. Observation helped one caregiver in his mid-forties notice a change in his lover:

> All of a sudden I'll take a good look at him and I notice how much weight he's losing. And I thought that he was beginning to lose weight again, and then coming back from the doctor yesterday, he confirmed it, that he had lost ten pounds.

Watching and analyzing often begins before the actual diagnosis of AIDS, when the person with AIDS shows symptoms that may be vague or unlabeled, such as a constant sore throat or slight fatigue. As time passes after diagnosis, some caregivers begin to feel more expert in interpreting subtle symptoms and comparing the sick person's experience to the "norm." Some family caregivers describe their watchfulness and wariness as using an imaginary antenna to "tune in" to the person with AIDS and monitor his or her ever-changing behavior.

However, no matter how much expertise they gain, analyzing information still poses a significant challenge for most caregivers. The symptoms of HIV can be complex, subtle, and confusing even to the most experienced caregiver. Since its appearance in the early 1980s, AIDS continues to manifest itself in bizarre ways. Even thrush, fatigue, loss of appetite, diarrhea and other common symptoms can present in an uncommon manner, and therefore can be difficult to understand. One man, who had brought his close friend with AIDS to his home to provide supervision and help, knew something was wrong:

> He was getting problems with digestion, and I tried all the normal things—you know, sleep on pillows, don't eat after a certain hour, cut down on fatty foods. I said, it's something other than the norm that I would follow with a normal person. So I took him in, and we discovered through ultrasound one of his glands was swollen and it was closing off his throat.

Caregivers often feel they cannot rely on persons with AIDS, especially children or people with mental impairment, to volunteer complete informa-

tion about how they feel. Instead, caregivers use both verbal and nonverbal communication to assess the sick person's condition. They observe the person with AIDS, watch for new symptoms, identify patterns, and actively question the person with AIDS about his or her health. A man in his thirties, caring for his lover of two years, said:

> He was having a hard time swallowing, and I said to him, "All right, you've got to really explain to me, like I can't see or hear." I said, "Draw me a picture of exactly what you're feeling."

Caregivers often become highly emotional when they notice a new symptom and realize its possible implications. A new cough may bring a response from a sense of dread to near-hysteria because it could indicate Pneumocystis pneumonia, a swift and possibly fatal AIDS-related disease. Even the mildest symptoms may be interpreted as "the tip of the iceberg," and cause caregivers a lot of anxiety.

"IS IT HIM OR THE DISEASE?"

As caregivers try to figure out what a symptom means, they face the major challenge of sorting emotional responses to the disease from the symptoms themselves. A sister noted:

You start seeing a lot of changes. The symptoms are very vague in the beginning, so you don't really know if this is stress, depression—or are there some clear signs, like his memory isn't what it used to be? At the same time, they have him on so much prednisone, he's having a lot of reaction to that. It's typical, but is it that or something else?

Caregivers fear they may overlook an important symptom by attributing it to the sick person's personality. They relentlessly examine each symptom for any sign that it could indicate a serious manifestation of the disease, such as a brain tumor, an opportunistic infection, or some milestone which suggests the beginning of a slow, steady deterioration.

Separating symptom from emotional response is more difficult when a caregiver feels AIDS has magnified the sick person's pre-AIDS personality traits. This young woman was part of a small group who shared the care of a close friend with AIDS:

You know, it's hard to tell, because he's a pretty far-out-there person anyway. It's, like, "Do you think he's crazy now? What do you guys think? I don't know." I mean, he goes out and buys a three hundred dollar funeral outfit. Is this crazy behavior? He's always done this. Maybe he's always been crazy! I guess

it doesn't matter, but I guess medically it matters if we think he needs to go to the hospital and he doesn't want to.

Many times, caregivers have to think on their feet and change their tactics for each new crisis. In the never-ending struggle to manage the constantly changing symptoms of HIV infection, caregivers in our study said they often would reuse or revise the strategy they used for the last symptom. If it didn't work, they would discard that strategy entirely and come up with other ideas.

"DOING FOR" *

Caregivers vary considerably in what and how much they do for the person with AIDS. The person with AIDS may have one symptom or many symptoms, not all of them disabling, and not all of them at once. "Doing for" usually involves performing tasks that persons with AIDS would do for themselves if they could, such as preparing meals or giving medicines. It's important to note that the person with AIDS doesn't need to be bedridden or extremely sick before "doing for" be-

---

*The language and concept of "Doing For" was influenced by Dr. Kristen Swanson's theory of caring, published in *Nursing Research*.

gins; much of caregiving is simply looking after household tasks that the sick person no longer has energy or mental strength to do.

Caregivers tailor what they do for a person with AIDS to what the sick person needs at the time. For example, caregivers of persons with fatigue may take over all of the housework chores. Caregivers of persons with mental impairment often assume responsibility for the sick person's personal business, such as managing money and completing insurance or state assistance forms. Mother caregivers may assume more of the sick person's personal care, since moms are often used to giving their children baths and cleaning up their messes. Also, features of the pre-AIDS relationship, such as who was "in charge," may determine the kinds of tasks the caregiver performs.

A caregiver provides different types of help, including:
(1) symptom management
(2) assisting with bathing, medications, safety, and other aspects of direct personal care
(3) managing the household and personal business, such as shopping and paying bills
(4) maintaining social activities, arranging visits and outings and keeping the sick person's friends and family informed
(5) interacting with the health care

system: participating in decision making and advocacy, and coordinating the person with AIDS's health care.

The mother of a young man with AIDS spoke of her day-to-day responsibilities:

The most important thing about all this is making sure that he eats well-balanced meals, and getting him up for exercise by walking around the block, and making sure he gets his medicines, trying to keep his mouth clean—it's a lot of little details.

Lack of guidance and information is a major obstacle for caregivers who are "doing for." They often have no guidelines to help them manage symptoms and make decisions about health care; they must learn by trial and error. Caregivers who lack access to information are likely to feel lost, as though they are "providing care in a vacuum." Previous experience with the care of others, such as an elderly parent or another person with AIDS, can help balance the difficulties of "doing for" and provide a useful foundation upon which to build caregiving skills and confidence. Also, sources of information such as support groups, home health nurses, friends who are also caregiving, and caregiver classes offer opportunities to share ideas for managing the illness. One thirty-eight-year-old father was particularly grateful for the opportunity to learn new information:

I didn't know what [caregiving] was all about until I went to this caregiving class at the Red Cross, and I'm glad I went, because I learned a lot. It really helped me to understand it.

Another challenge of "doing for" is called "fighting the wasting." Wasting away, weight loss, and general physical deterioration are inescapable visual reminders of AIDS, and caregivers, such as this wife, make controlling them an urgent priority:

I think the biggest thing, besides the emotional side of it, has been food. The thrush makes food taste bad and the medication makes food taste worse, and he's lost thirty pounds, and so we've tried to find ways of keeping his weight up. I try to find things that taste good, or try to keep mealtime a less emotional time, so he will eat. We've got him on a weight-gain body building thing to drink in between eating sessions. It's a challenge for me to find things that taste good to him. A lot of his favorite things don't taste good anymore, and anything that requires much chewing he just can't handle.

Malnutrition, muscle wasting, and starvation are themselves life-threatening conditions; consequently, the drastic weight loss so common to persons with AIDS often makes grocery shopping, food preparation, and coaching the person with AIDS to eat seem like crucial and significant matters. One twenty-two-year-old man caring for his lover found that this was one of the most difficult parts of caregiving:

Right now the biggest problem is trying to get him to eat. He has long periods when he has no appetite. If he doesn't eat, he'll lose more, and faster. Neither of us has ever been domestic in this regard. Neither of us can cook, and suddenly it becomes urgent to have food in the house and get food eaten.

Caregivers reported several strategies they used to fight the wasting: making food more appealing, making food accessible, catering to whims, cajoling and encouraging the person with AIDS to eat, forcing foods, and monitoring the person with AIDS's nutritional intake. They also spoke of "tricks of the trade" they had learned from nurses and dieticians to add extra calories to food, such as mixing an instant breakfast powder into a milkshake.

Since food is associated with nurturing, the caregiver's attempts to feed the sick person and fight the wasting have additional symbolism. The image of someone carefully carrying a bowl of steaming soup to a bedridden person is an icon in our culture; it means that even though the person in the bed is ill, he or she is safe, warm, and loved. Feeding the sick person can make the caregiver feel good, too. It's a tangible sign of the caregiver's love and concern, and it can have visible results: the sick person maintains or puts on weight.

"Doing for" is not always straightforward. Caregivers struggle with uncertainty and self-doubt as they wonder how much they should help the person with AIDS, how to deal with refusals from the person with AIDS, whether they should encourage the person with AIDS to do things for himself or herself, and how best to motivate the person with AIDS in self-care. The needs of a person with AIDS can fluctuate, and caregivers often fear they will make mistakes. Also, caregivers may have to deal with criticism or conflicting advice from friends about choices they make for the person with AIDS. One woman was uncertain whether to cater to the food preferences of her friend with AIDS, or listen to her nutrition-minded friends:

> And I made a list, and I was, like, "I'm gonna go shopping. We're going to get you some of these." He was telling me,

give me canned syrupy peaches, and all this stuff. And all these health-conscious people freaked out. They're going, "Twinkies! Oh, my God! Don't feed him those!"

COORDINATING HELP

Caregivers often want relief from their caregiving activities, or they may eventually reach a point of overload when they realize they can't continue to "go it alone." It is rare that one individual can provide everything a person with AIDS needs: caregivers need concrete help and support from others. They may seek assistance from professional home care services or volunteer errand services, or from their own and the sick person's family and social networks. Caregivers often arrange to have other people give the person with AIDS something the caregiver cannot provide, such as transportation to medical appointments while the caregiver is at work. A caregiver may also wish to hire assistance such as a housecleaning service in order to have time for his or her personal activities.

However, asking for help doesn't ensure that caregivers will get what they need or want. A lesbian caregiver, part of a group of women that took care of a close friend with AIDS, found this out from experience:

In a way it's been really nice to get help from my mother, but I'm also a little cautious, too. I've been let down by so many people that I don't let everybody know how caregiving is affecting me. I keep lots to myself, and on occasion would ask support from her. I also knew there was only so much she could give.

Coordinating help is a hidden part of managing the illness, since it isn't a direct care activity. Yet, it usually requires a lot of the caregiver's time and energy to organize assistance from others. It may be jointly accomplished with the person with AIDS, or tinged with conflict and resistance from the person with AIDS. Caregivers may need to solicit help despite the sick person's protests. Some persons with AIDS strongly prefer to accept only the family caregiver's help; others are reluctant to accept help from anyone.

A caregiver usually becomes the primary communicator of the person with AIDS's condition to the rest of the world, particularly as the person with AIDS becomes more ill or less able to interact. A thirty-year-old gay man told how his role as care manager for his lover evolved into that of spokesman:

That comes with the consistency of being there. They start to realize that I've been there every time he's been sick, and I've managed the house, and I've managed

his health care, and whenever he was in the hospital I was their contact to find out what was going on, that I was on top of things.

This knowledgeable role affects caregivers in different ways. On one hand, caregivers are sometimes worn out by the stress of explaining again and again the sick person's condition. The caregiver may return home exhausted from the hospital, only to find messages on the answering machine from the sick person's parents, sister, best friend, lawyer—all wanting immediate updates. On the other hand, some caregivers find relief in "unloading" and talking to someone about their ordeal, especially if the person who asks is sensitive enough to inquire about the caregiver's well-being, too.

The family caregiver may notice that the person with AIDS is unwilling or unable to ask for needed support or companionship. In these situations, coordinating help involves activating the sick person's network of friends and family. One middle-aged man saw his partner's spirits improve when friends called, so he made sure that happened:

I go through his phone book finding phone numbers and saying, "Hey, Paul needs a lift. I think if you called him he'd really perk up."

COMMUNICATING WITH HEALTH CARE PROFESSIONALS

Even in times of relative well-being, most persons with AIDS want the caregiver to be included in meetings with health care professionals. Caregivers often play a key role in identifying problems and getting appropriate treatment because they've watched the person with AIDS so closely. For instance, some caregivers we interviewed noticed that persons with AIDS minimized their symptoms when they described them later to health care professionals, and insisted that they felt fine. It's often up to the caregiver to tell the professional how things *really* are—how many times the person with AIDS threw up the night before, how much pain the sick person seemed to suffer.

A thirty-six-year-old musical instrument maker felt that even though he is not a health care professional, his ideas enhanced his lover's care:

I want the best possible care for my partner. I had to suggest giving him physical therapy.

However, in a health care system which is almost exclusively aimed at the individual patient, many family caregivers feel they are a vital source of information untapped by professional care providers. Caregivers who think professionals are ignoring them and missing important information often fight to be heard, and challenge decisions the professionals have made. Family caregivers often try to negotiate a partnership with professionals, or change doctors if they don't feel they can work with the one they have been seeing. In time, most professionals realize the value of the family caregiver and start to rely on him or her for specific information or an overall assessment of the sick person's condition.

BEING MANAGED BY THE ILLNESS

A middle-aged woman described the constant demands of caring for her husband:

He's tired all the time, he can't make his own food half the time, and he gets sick like that, and when he does, whether he's in the hospital or not, it takes constant brainpower. You're constantly thinking and worrying about him, and having to bring him things, and help him speak with the doctors, and just work everything out.

Relentless day-to-day caregiving activities can take their toll on a caregiver. Although it's the caregiver's job to keep the illness in a manageable state and treat each new symptom as it arises, the caregiver isn't always the one in command. Sometimes it's as if the tables are turned, and the illness has taken complete control of the caregiver's life. The pain of loss, the pressures of the relationship between caregiver and care-receiver, and the stigma and potential danger of HIV, joined with all the mental, physical, and emotional work of managing the sick person's illness on a daily basis, make the caregiver feel as if he or she is being managed by AIDS. One middle-aged teacher caring for his lover felt his life was consumed by AIDS caregiving:

Other people who are in a caregiving situation in a hospital can shut it off after eight hours. I can't ever shut it off; I have no way of ever shutting it off. I'm not sure I'd wish to if I could—but I have to live with it twenty- four hours a day, seven days a week. If there were only some way of getting other folks to cross that threshold and see what it's like: that there is no easy way of doing this.

While the extent to which the family caregiver is consumed by managing the illness depends on the style of the caregiver as well as the needs of the person with AIDS, most people experience considerable strain from the demands of caregiving, as this lover of a person with AIDS noted:

I call it "going out and feeling sorry for myself." It sounds really self-centered, but, yeah, there are a lot of things in my life that are not very good right now— you know, involved with his illness. It bothers the heck out of me. It makes me very sad and very angry.

For some caregivers, the cumulative stress may result in burnout that seriously hampers the caregiver's quality of life, as this man caring for his long-time lover said:

[Caregiving] is the hardest thing I have ever done in my life. Nothing even prepared me for this. Sometimes I wonder if I'll ever recover.

Despite the enormous amount of work a caregiver does to manage the illness, the helpless feeling of "never being able to do enough" contributes to the perception of being managed. A thirty-year-old man struggled to maintain his work as a bank teller while being "on duty" day and night to help his lover:

He went into hysterics and I couldn't calm him down, and I finally made the decision that we were going to the hospital, and I stayed with him for twelve whole hours in the emergency room while they decided what they were going to do with him. Then they didn't have a bed available, so I took him back home and waited twenty-four hours and they finally had a space for him so I brought him back. That forty-eight hours was probably the worst I've spent yet, and I told him I wouldn't leave him, and in fact at one point I had to call work because I hadn't had any sleep and I was gonna try to get about two hours and then go back into work.

Many people find it difficult to assume complete responsibility for someone else's life and well-being. However, a family caregiver may want and need to be involved extensively in the sick person's care, even though it means relinquishing his or her own independence for a length of time. Some consider their being managed by the illness a sacrifice they're willing to make for someone they care for deeply. One stepfather was ready to make the sacrifice again:

There's nothing easy about it. But I don't begrudge it. If any of my other kids had it, I'd do the same thing for them. I'd be there.

INDEPENDENT CARE DECISIONS

A person with AIDS's need for assistance varies throughout the illness. At times, it's possible for the sick person to handle some of his or her own care. Some caregivers choose to leave certain decisions to the person with AIDS—for instance, how and when to take medications.

However, during episodes of acute illness or mental impairment, or during the terminal phase, caregivers may feel it's important to take complete control of the sick person's care. Depression, reduced mental ability, anorexia, and lethargy—several of the most common problems associated with AIDS—make it risky to rely exclusively on the person with AIDS for vigilant self-monitoring. Family members learn through experience that persons with mental impairment often can't be relied upon to take care of themselves. One man described the frightening experience of finding his lover at home, critically ill:

He was in his apartment and he was very, very sick and he was in a lot of denial. And the reality of it was that he was developing cryptococcal meningitis. And he was becoming demented and totally out of it. He would drop the phone and not pick it up, and stuff like that. I'd be screaming into the phone and there'd be no answer, and then I would hang up. Finally I said, "I think you've got to go into the hospital." I went to pick him up, and he had difficulty buzzing me into the apartment. When I got into the apartment, it was a total mess. There was rotting food all over. And driving him to the hospital, he was totally out of it. He didn't know who he was. They actually did not expect him to live.

Therefore, caregivers are often unwilling to take chances in letting the person with AIDS make independent care decisions. A sister emphasized how she was taking over more and more:

So now I've told him, and I've told all my neighbors and friends, I swear if he even coughs you take him to the doctor right away. Don't let him decide. That's gonna be our policy from now on.

Eventually, during the final stages of the disease, persons with AIDS depend entirely on family members to manage their whole world at home.

THINGS TO THINK ABOUT

- It's hard to know if you're doing the "right thing" to manage your loved one's illness. However, as time goes on, you'll gain experience and feel more confident.

- Sometimes, despite your best efforts, the person with AIDS may get worse. Don't be too hard on yourself if you can't control all the symptoms of AIDS or all of the effects of the disease.

- "Fighting the wasting" may consume a lot of time and energy. Even if the ill person loses weight, your efforts to provide good food still symbolize your love and nurturing.

- Don't be surprised if the question "Is it him, or the disease?" surfaces again and again. Mental impairment in the ill person is particularly hard to figure out.

- Find which resources are available in your community. Use them to save yourself time and keep yourself from burning out. Some assistance is free, while other services may cost money. Call your local AIDS hotline for more information.

- You have a lot to offer doctors, nurses, and social workers that can help them do a better job. If your loved one wants you to be involved, insist that professionals listen to you.

- Taking care of yourself is a wise investment. In the long run, you will be a better caregiver if you don't neglect your own needs.

- Realize that you may not be able to keep up with the demands of caregiving indefinitely. If the strain is too much, it can be just as loving to consider other options for the sick person, such as round-the-clock nurses or an AIDS house or hospice.

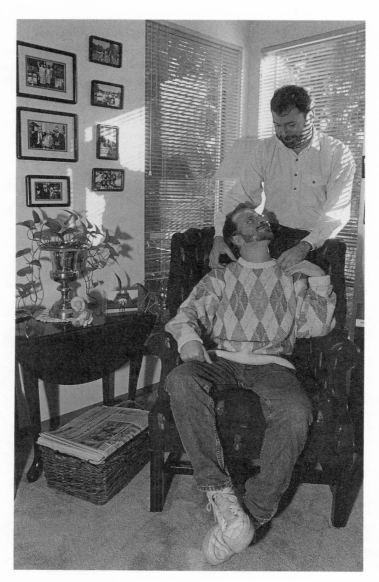

"When one person needs support, the other one is there, and it's been a two-way street. I get as much out of this relationship as I give. I guess that's the part of being in a relationship—the more you give, the more you get out of it."

Renegotiating the Relationship

The bottom line of family caregiving is a relationship between two people. Usually, they know each other well before the onset of AIDS. However, these people often find that the new roles of caregiver and care-receiver have thrust them into uncharted territory. They must understand each other on new terms, rethinking their roles and renegotiating the give-and-take of daily life. And, since AIDS can change people in unpredictable ways, caregivers who met the person with AIDS after the illness began must also renegotiate how they will relate to each other from day to day.

Renegotiation may be intentional or unconscious, smooth or full of conflict. How it happens depends on the current health and emotional well-being of the person with AIDS as well as the emotional well-being of the caregiver. A gay man caring for his lover commented:

> Our relationship has grown since [the AIDS diagnosis]. I think it's constantly growing and evolving, which is what I guess they say about all relationships. The relationship is definitely going through a change right now. Matt has been ill, and he is starting to grasp the reality that he may not be here very much longer.

In this chapter, caregivers describe how AIDS has changed their relationship with the sick person, and what's involved in the process of renegotiating the relationship.

TAKING ON THE CAREGIVER ROLE

In the beginning, people are likely to form tentative images of themselves as family caregivers, and of the journey they're about to take. They ask themselves, "How will I do this? How involved will I be?"—questions that will continue during the course of caregiving. They consider their resources, and how much they are prepared to give of themselves.

However, as they begin caregiving, very few people really understand the responsibilities and experiences that accompany this endeavor. They take on the role, later to face unforeseeable duties and hardships. This may lead them to reassess their abilities, which in turn can have a significant impact on what they will do for the person with AIDS.

MODIFYING GIVE AND TAKE

Like any relationship, family caregiving is a transaction; a mutual exchange takes place between two people. People who are closely involved expect things from one another in day-to-day life, and expect to give something in return, whether it's emotional support, shared housework, financial assistance, or countless other favors. A caregiver who is also the lover of the person in his care put it this way:

When one person needs support, the other one is there, and it's been a two-way street. I get as much out of this relationship as I give. I guess that's the part of being in a relationship—the more you give, the more you get out of it.

However, the illness may force the person with AIDS to give up his or her end of the bargain as energy and strength wane. Caregivers modify reciprocity, or "give and take," by adjusting the balance of favors and privileges within the relationship. A caregiver in his late forties, who brought his lover to live with him after an illness crisis, discussed the effect AIDS has had in their lives:

It distorts the relationship which is important to you, and which is in many instances built on a kind of reciprocity— whatever balance you might have worked out. It's quite altered in ways that might not have been your choice.

The health and the functional ability of the person with AIDS influence the caregiver's sense of how much to give and how much to take. When an acute illness crisis strikes, caregivers are likely to focus strictly on the sick person's needs and relinquish their own. During calm periods in the sick person's health, caregivers are more likely to value reciprocity once again and expect a more balanced give-and-take relationship.

While renegotiating the relationship mainly concerns the caregiver and the person with AIDS, renegotiation can extend to other relationships as well. Caregivers who aren't coupled with the person with AIDS, such as parents or friends, must renegotiate with their own primary partners, friends, and families in order to accommodate the caregiving role. The mother of a twenty-two-year-old man with AIDS worked out a routine with her husband, the sick person's stepfather:

Me and my husband take turns going places. My husband went out last night, and today he's going to get his hair cut, and it's my day to stay at home. Tomor-row I get to run the streets, go shop-ping, then tomorrow night we're going to a birthday party so my mother is go-ing to come stay here. We get someone to come in and look after him, then we get a chance to do something together. But, it's been really hard on our mar-riage. I could see the stress this could put on a marriage, if people aren't strong.

TAKING CARE OF YOURSELF

As much as some caregivers wish to be selfless, it's very difficult to sus-pend completely your own physical and emotional needs: as one caregiver put it, "We're not Mother Theresas." The contradiction between altruistic in-tentions and human needs of caregiv-ers surfaces quite often. A caregiver may be reluctant to take care of him-self or herself, as this lover of a person with AIDS noted:

I feel guilty because I need time away. That is a bit much, you know, after you spend three days straight with him. I feel guilty lots of times when he's not feeling well and [I make] a choice to go out and do something for myself. But it's at a point that I really do feel I need some space.

The desire to please the person with AIDS at all costs can keep the caregiver from even considering that his or her own needs may be as important as the sick person's care. However, most fam-ily members who remain in the role of caregiver eventually learn how to care for themselves while caring for a per-son with AIDS. Support groups and counseling, caregiver courses, and en-couragement from close friends can confirm the legitimacy of the caregiver's attention to his or her personal needs, even those that might contradict the wishes of the person with AIDS. A middle-aged man taking care of his lover described how he handled this problem:

In our support group people have gotten into hassles with their sick lovers because the lover doesn't want strangers coming into the house, and I'm really strong in presenting the view that you just tell the person, "Well, I'm doing it because I need the assistance. I can't clean the house, and the person is going to come in to help me with this problem —it has nothing to do with you. I don't need your permission to decide whether I should wash the kitchen floor, or study for my exams that are coming up, or deal with my business, or whatever."

GETTING SUPPORT FROM THE PERSON WITH AIDS

If the caregiving relationship is indeed a two-way street, how much support may the caregiver appropriately expect from the person in his or her care? Most caregivers eventually become comfortable expecting something from the person with AIDS, unless the person with AIDS is quite mentally or physically debilitated. One type of support caregivers may want is concrete assistance; for instance, they may ask the person with AIDS to do the laundry while the caregiver is at work.

Other caregivers may want the person with AIDS not to do tasks, and instead save the precious commodity of energy for activities with the caregiver. Honoring these requests can become a sensitive issue in relationships, and conflicts may arise when the person with AIDS ignores them. For example, the caregiver may feel betrayed when the person with AIDS overexerts doing household chores in order to feel "useful," and is then too exhausted to enjoy activities with the caregiver.

A caregiver usually wants to feel that the person with AIDS is grateful for the work he or she is doing; in fact, gratitude from the person with AIDS is an especially important type of support our caregivers mentioned. Unless the person with AIDS is significantly disabled, caregivers often expect the person with AIDS to treat them well—to speak kindly, and to try to understand the caregiver's point of view. Caregivers in our study wanted common expressions of caring, such as appreciation, listening, emotional support, and interest in their activities and well-being.

The sick person's expression of concern can be a notable reward. One caregiver in his twenties who was caring for his partner of seven years felt frustrated and hurt without that attention:

> I had a lot of things to tell him, all the things that had been going on while I was gone, and he wasn't responsive like I wanted him to be. You know, I wanted feedback. I wanted to hear whether I did something right or wrong, and I just wasn't getting it. I'm not sure if he was really listening, and that's happening a lot more these days.

COPING WITH DEPENDENCY

The ability to rely on another person for help or support is a vital component of close relationships. In caregiving, however, this reliance becomes more intense and less reciprocal. As the sick person's dependency on the caregiver increases, their connection can start to resemble a parent-to-child relationship. One caregiver, who had already raised a teenage son, felt reluctant to go through the same experience with his sick lover:

Having been a single parent for all these years, I did not want another situation where it's like having another kid, which of course it is. And that's been difficult.

Increased dependency is difficult because it may diminish the self-respect of the person with AIDS, increase the burden of responsibility on the caregiver, and erode the pre-existing patterns of give and take in the relationship. Even parents caring for a younger child with AIDS may feel overwhelmed by the additional dependency that accompanies a terminal illness.

The amount of dependency shifts with the ill person's health. Children with AIDS who aren't feeling well may want to be held more. Adults with AIDS may simply want the caregiver to be more accessible. Certain manifestations of AIDS, such as mental impairment, may take away whatever independence the sick person has and greatly increase his or her need for constant care. The parent of a young man with AIDS who lives with him noted the extra attention a person with mental disability needs:

You can't leave him alone too long, because you never know how the mind's going to be. Like, one time I went to sleep, and I thought he was in his room, and he had checked himself back into the hospital.

Caregivers are usually willing to accept more responsibility during heightened illness, and to put work, school, or other relationships on hold while they devote themselves completely to the person with AIDS. As the sick person's health improves, most caregivers are willing or eager to let go of some of this responsibility, and let the person with AIDS do as much self-care as possible until the next illness crisis.

Dependency can cause tension between the caregiver and the person with AIDS as they try to work together to manage the illness. A caregiver may become frustrated with the sick person's unwillingness or refusal to accept help. One woman struggled with her need to please her partner:

I work very hard on something, and it doesn't taste good to him, and I'm just angry at the situation. You try to give him some good information, or something the doctor has said, and they don't want to hear it. You're trying to do the right thing for them, and sometimes nothing is right. It's frustrating.

To balance both their own and the sick person's discomfort with dependency, caregivers often attempt to foster independence in the person with AIDS. In fact, some caregivers invest considerable energy to make sure that the person with AIDS can continue self-care for as long as possible. One lover noted:

> I'm letting him deal with [taking medicines]. You have to be real subtle and sensitive. They say it's an important thing for him to take medicines at the right time and so forth, but it's almost as important for him to be in control as much as possible.

When true independence is impossible, some caregivers attempt to create the illusion of independence. They may even deceive the people in their care to protect them from humiliation or physical harm and to reduce the impact of dependency without compromising their care and safety. This bank officer, accustomed to being in charge at work, outwardly relinquished control in order to help his partner feel more independent:

> Even though I let him be in charge of his medicines, I knew what was going on with each one. I checked up on him without letting him know by counting his pills.

MINIMIZING CONFLICT

Relationships, especially intimate ones, are rarely smooth. Struggle and conflict are inevitable as two individuals create and maintain an environment which affects them both. The challenges and difficulties of having AIDS and caring for someone with AIDS can accelerate conflicts in a relationship. The stress of AIDS can especially aggravate pre-existing issues or conflicts, as this caregiver, a political science graduate student, noted:

> AIDS exaggerates people. Every kind of emotion or feeling is magnified; whatever kind of idiosyncrasies you have ever had are magnified. One of Rob's is an abandonment thing; I'm not exactly sure where that comes from, perhaps his last relationship he was in before me. And so it seems like there have been times since he's had AIDS where what I think are real innocuous things have become big for him. I think, "Who is this person? Why didn't I know about this before?"

Friction between the caregiver and the person with AIDS can become more intense as pressures accompanying the illness escalate and patience decreases. Caregivers can become unhappy with certain facets of the sick person's behavior toward them. They may feel the person in their care tries to manipulate or take advantage of them. One young woman caring for a friend wrestled with the problem of where to draw the line with him:

I think he can do more when I'm not there. Often he won't eat, and it feels a bit manipulative, just because that's a role that's played between the two of us.

However, the knowledge that the person with AIDS may soon be gone often motivates caregivers to minimize conflicts and resolve differences peacefully. And, sometimes, sheer exhaustion or the need to preserve his or her own energy causes the caregiver to defer to the person with AIDS.

Caregivers note that they become more patient; they're more likely to give in to the person with AIDS during an argument and let go of resentments that arise. They may choose not to become angry, not to express negative feelings to the person with AIDS, not to point out the sick person's irritating behavior. Flexibility, tolerance, and forgiveness become important tools for minimizing conflict. A caregiver in his forties, the lover of the person with AIDS, understood this well:

You have to deal with aspects of [the relationship] in a way that doesn't allow some of the techniques that you might use with a more healthy person in a re-

lationship. You have to tolerate it and work around it.

A common strategy caregivers use to keep the peace is carefully "choosing battles." Some things they might have argued about in the past are no longer worth the struggle; caregivers decide which issues are important enough to fight over and which can be let go. This new approach to negotiation helps the caregiver consider which topics to avoid, how best to speak to the person with AIDS, and when to defer to the person with AIDS during an argument.

Choosing battles also means excusing the person with AIDS for his or her less-than-desirable behavior. Caregivers work hard to understand how difficult life must be for the person with AIDS. They often regard the sick person's unkind words or self-centered behavior as reactions to the illness, and they try to help others have a similarly accepting attitude. This outlook seems particularly important when the person with AIDS has some illness-related mental damage and unexplained behavior. One mother tried to help her husband cope with these symptoms:

My husband gets real frustrated with our son, and I have to remind him that Bob is not himself, so it's not his fault that he's like that.

A caregiver may feel an urgent need to get along well with the person with AIDS, and to interact with him or her in a positive way. With careful management, conflicts may be replaced with a new sense of teamwork and harmony within the relationship, as this gay man observed:

> Our relationship was very good in lots of ways, but [caregiving] has heightened and developed and strengthened the relationship. A lot of it is very poignant and very beautiful and very bittersweet.

Minimizing conflict and maintaining harmony within the relationship is not without its costs. These costs become more apparent to caregivers as the person with AIDS becomes sicker or as the duration of caregiving increases. Caregivers may begin to feel resentful and angry about constantly having to accommodate the person with AIDS and keep the peace. However, caregivers are usually reluctant to show their anger to the people in their care, so they find other ways to deal with it. Many caregivers find support group meetings and caregiving classes outlets for communicating their frustration. Others may suppress their feelings, expressing them through physical symptoms such as headaches or ulcers, or taking them out on people in their other relationships.

ABANDONING THE CAREGIVER ROLE

For some caregivers, the relationship with the person with AIDS may become so uncomfortable that they eventually decide to abandon the caregiver role, or place the sick person in an institution. And, it is important to note that some people are unwilling or unable to become a primary family caregiver. Even for those who actively assume the caregiving role, the question of whether to remain in this role may resurface periodically. Although most of the caregivers reported that they intended to continue with caregiving until the sick person's death, a small number considered leaving the role before then. For these people, the costs of the relationship outweighed the motivation to stay.

Some people caring for lovers were rejected by family members who didn't approve of the sick person's homosexuality or drug use. Others found that the relationship they had with the person with AIDS before diagnosis just wasn't strong enough to withstand the added strain of illness. Some caregivers couldn't cope with the sick person's emotional responses to the illness or the symptoms of HIV, especially mental impairment. One man decided to leave his partner because staying with her simply became too difficult:

They said they were going to release her [from the psychiatric ward of the hospital], and I said, "Okay, but if you guys are going to release her, then I have to tell you I don't think that I've had enough time away from her where I feel well. I don't think I feel safe around her because of her violence and rage. I do feel fear. Therefore, I'm going to have to take the initiative and choose to not be around her any more." I said good-bye, good luck—I took off down the street.

Caregiving is a tough job for everyone involved, and it can be difficult to keep a relationship together through the incredible strain of life-threatening illness. Caregivers find it helps to anticipate potential problems, to choose battles carefully, to recognize that increased conflict often reflects a normal reaction to the stress and fear of their situation, and to live one day at a time.

THINGS TO THINK ABOUT

- Changes in your relationship with the ill person are inevitable as his or her health changes. Old expectations and patterns of being together may not work any more. Develop new ways of relating to each other. For example, give your loved one more slack, but don't let him or her take advantage of you.
- Sometimes the sick person may forget that you have needs, too. It's okay to remind the person with AIDS about things that are important to you.

- It's natural to want appreciation from your loved one for all the things you do. Let him or her know that a "thank you" can go a long way. Seek affirmation from other family members and friends; let them know it's important to feel appreciated.

- The amount of help the sick person needs from you will ebb and flow. These changes can be difficult, and will require you to shift the amount of responsibility you assume. Remember that persons with AIDS may lose some self-respect when others do for them what they used to be able to do for themselves.

- You and your loved one are under stress, and conflict is natural and likely under these circumstances. "Choosing your battles" can help you keep the peace without sacrificing what is important to you.

- It's natural to question your commitment to caregiving—it's part of the response to the difficulties that may occur. Ultimately, it is your right to decide whether you feel able to take care of your loved one.

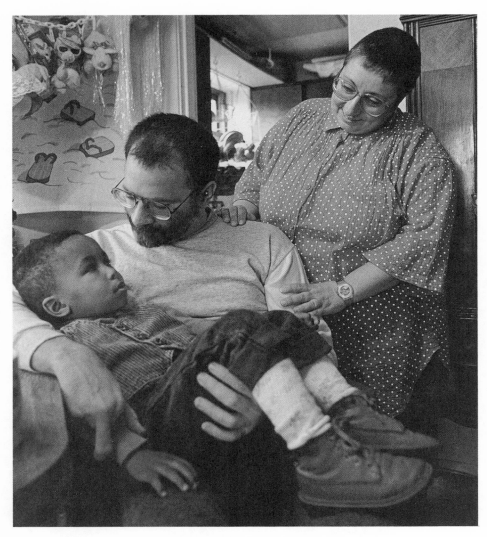

"My story is an open book. I don't feel like I have anything to hide from anybody about this subject. There is such a conspiracy of silence. I hate that."

Going Public

Suddenly, it's official: the doctor has confirmed the diagnosis of AIDS. Now, the sick person faces two principal issues. First, although medicines are available to relieve some of the symptoms, the disease itself has no cure. Second, for the rest of his or her life, he or she is marked as a "person with AIDS," a term that will change the lives of both the sick person and the caregiver.

Deciding who, when, and how to tell someone that you are an AIDS caregiver can be difficult. Is it possible to keep it a secret? When is it better to tell someone? In this chapter, family caregivers discuss the benefits and drawbacks of going public as an AIDS caregiver.

THE PROBLEM OF AIDS STIGMA

Many in our society connect AIDS and the people who have it with crime, failure, and weakness. Since family caregivers are the people most closely associated with the person with AIDS, caregivers also find themselves targets of AIDS phobia and negative judgment.

One caregiver summarized this fact with bitterness: "People feel like AIDS is a dirty disease and people associate it with dirty people no matter what." This "guilt by association" explains why AIDS stigma emerged from our study as a significant concern of family caregivers. Both the person with AIDS and the caregiver are called into question because of society's discomfort with sexuality (particularly homosexuality), and drug abuse.

However, AIDS stigma wasn't reported only by caregivers of persons with AIDS who were drug users or homosexuals. People taking care of persons with AIDS who contracted HIV by "socially acceptable" routes, such as blood transfusion, also experienced the ostracism caused by fear of contagion and death. Even though HIV is only spread through direct contact with body fluids or shared needles, the terror of catching the disease through everyday contact has cost some persons with AIDS and their caregivers their jobs, friends, and homes.

LIVING WITH SECRECY

Telling people you're an AIDS family caregiver can be a risky move. It's often difficult to know how people will react to the news. Are they informed about the low risk of contracting AIDS from everyday contact, or do they know nothing about AIDS except the terror of getting it? Will they understand the importance of caregiving and the challenges you face, or will they suddenly decide it's better never to see you again?

To protect themselves and the persons with AIDS from harm, a number of caregivers in the survey kept their caregiving a secret. They pretended they weren't AIDS caregivers, or they were very careful with the information that they were caring for a family member with AIDS. A forty-five-year-old wife caregiver discussed her reasons for living with secrecy:

There are a lot of people you can go to, but they would have very strong feelings about him and they would tell you what a really rotten person he is, and what in the hell are you doing staying there in that household? And they'd be very fearful of you getting the disease. I just couldn't handle anybody else's judgement, anybody else's anger, anybody else's fear.

The caregivers in our study were often afraid information about their caregiver role would discredit them among family members, friends, neighbors, work colleagues, and acquaintances. Some of the more open caregivers discovered this firsthand; they reported that after going public they had been harassed and rejected, and that they had lost jobs, friends, and housing. One caregiver, a supermarket employee, chose secrecy to safeguard his job:

I was told by my boss about seven or eight months ago that if I told any of the employees that Rob has AIDS I would be fired.

To be safe, another told his landlord only part of the truth:

The landlord doesn't know the whole situation. He knows that Linda is very sick, but he doesn't know what's wrong with us, that we're both HIV positive and that she's got all these things wrong with her.

Many caregivers said they suffered greatly from shame, fear of disclosure and repercussions, and ridicule and negative judgement from others. A partner caregiver, who hadn't told her family that she was caring for someone with AIDS, expressed her anger about pervasive anti-AIDS sentiment:

It's people's ignorance of AIDS and their cruelty with the disease that makes it really hard. I mean, you listen to jokes all the time about AIDS. Like at our Thanksgiving dinner, everybody had a different joke about AIDS.

Jokes and disparaging comments about AIDS hit one father caregiver especially hard:

When I found out my son had AIDS, I was at work one day. Like I said, no one knows my son's got AIDS but two people, and there were a bunch of guys joking about it, about AIDS, you know. I got so pissed I took a table and just slammed it on the floor and walked out. It got to me that much, guys joking, and they looked at me like I was crazy. I just picked up the table and dropped it on the floor and turned around and walked out because it got to me. I got tired of hearing about queers and AIDS. They were making jokes about people with AIDS, and I really got tired of that, but they don't know why I dropped the table. I never told them.

Caregivers reported that in order to keep their secret they lied, made excuses, withheld information, changed jobs or places of residence, and avoided certain social situations, such as family gatherings. Many of them used several of these strategies at the same time. One partner caregiver found the best way to keep his secret was to avoid people

as much as possible:

The people that are probably closest to me know that there has been problems. I haven't gone much further than that. They haven't been demanding and asking a lot of questions, and have accepted my very brief explanation, but you stay away from people.

Secrecy often resulted in a web of selective disclosure filled with lies, partial truths, and excuses. The set of complex ruses frequently became a source of great emotional turmoil. Caregivers were afraid they'd say the wrong thing, or that they'd contradict what they had said previously. One wife whose husband refused to tell their teenage children that he had AIDS felt the constant burden of deceit and the fear of discovery. She was angry about how this dishonesty hindered closeness with her children, and she felt frustrated about the considerable energy required to remember and juggle information. She worried constantly about what she said to whom as she struggled to create plausible and consistent excuses:

I have to keep some of his schedule a secret. We see a lot of doctors, and sometimes he'll have to have a lot of tests. It's covering up with the kids where I have to ask myself, "What did I just tell them last week?" Try to remember the same excuse.

STAGING INFORMATION

When secretive caregivers decided to share the fact that they were AIDS family caregivers, they usually staged information disclosure and increased the amount of information given over time. They carefully selected a certain amount and type of information and slowly painted a complete picture. One longtime lover, an office worker, became adept at selectively sharing and staging information with his co-workers:

There's been days where I have taken off from work and I've told people there, not being specific, that I have a sick person living with me. I refer to him as my nephew, that he is ill, and he does have a terminal illness.

In most cases, staging information involved: 1) simply talking about a sick friend or family member, regardless of the actual relationship, 2) elaborating that the person had a serious illness other than AIDS or was dying, and 3) finally sharing the explicit diagnosis of AIDS, their relationship to the person with AIDS, and the extent of their caregiving role.

One man caring for his lover ran into trouble when his parents pressured him to come home for a visit. He hadn't yet reached the final stages of sharing the information:

My parents know I have a friend who is sick. I was supposed to come back east on some work just about a year ago, and I had to cancel that trip. They were very disappointed, and I had to give them a reason why. I told them I had a sick friend, and also that this sick friend of mine now lives in the house and that he needed a place to live. They don't know that he's still sick. They think that he just had meningitis. So it's an uncomfortable set of ruses.

Generally, the sick person's health status affects decisions about the timing and staging of disclosure. Heightened illness often forces increased openness; as the person with AIDS becomes sicker, the caregiver discloses more information about the situation to more people. Other times people become more assertive are after the diagnosis of AIDS, or during a hospitalization or serious illness episode. A mother, who during the interview was very sad and tearful about her son's deteriorating condition, related:

When I started on this job I didn't tell them, because I don't just say, "Oh, hi, how are you? My son has AIDS," you know? I didn't tell them because I didn't see the need to, but then as I saw Benny getting sick I told them something was going on.

However, as AIDS progresses, physical changes can make it impossible to keep the disease a secret. One caregiver realized that the person she was caring for couldn't lose much more weight before people would have to be told:

Now it's coming to the point where—like, I've gotten out of work to take him to some of these tests and things, and of course they want to know what's wrong, and it's a whole bunch of lies. He's lost enough weight now that everybody has been saying, "Oh, gosh, he's just looking so good!" because everybody over fifty is overweight and wants to lose weight, and here he is getting nice and trim.

LIVING OPENLY

Some caregivers in our study didn't need to stage information or keep their caregiving a secret. Some chose to ignore the AIDS stigma and live openly in their caregiving role from the beginning. One woman, whose life partner was a hemophiliac with AIDS, asserted her involvement with AIDS in every dimension of her life. Together they had made numerous media appearances, and felt both pride in their community education efforts and anger about others' secrecy:

My story is an open book. I don't feel

like I have anything to hide from anybody about this subject. There is such a conspiracy of silence. I hate that.

Some assertive caregivers we spoke to had become activists committed to ending the social oppression of those affected by AIDS and AIDS stigma. They worked toward change in economic and political structures, including social and health care policies and cultural beliefs related to HIV infection. They wanted to demonstrate self-pride and affirm a belief that they could change society's responses to people with HIV infection. Some caregivers routinely monitored the media for the accuracy of AIDS-related information, wrote letters to authors to correct inaccurate statements and dispel myths, or appeared on television to promote AIDS education and prevention. One man was enraged by a syndicated newspaper columnist's advice which bore the headline "Never, Never, Never Have Sex With a Person With AIDS." This caregiver wrote a response to the columnist that was subsequently published, and said he expressed righteous anger in this excerpt from his letter:

We are a gay couple....Your statement that no one should have sex with an AIDS patient seems wrong to us. Sexual practices like mutual masturbation and frottage have never transmitted AIDS to anyone. You should tell this to people. AIDS patients are human beings and need sexual expression: People who love AIDS patients may want to express that love physically. This goes for gays and heterosexuals equally. "Having sex" is not necessarily having intimate contact with body fluids: I should not have to point that out to a sex expert.

How open a person had been about AIDS-related factors such as homosexuality or drug use before he or she began caring for a person with AIDS often determines how secretive or outspoken he or she is as a caregiver. For example, a mother caregiver who previously had discussed her son's homosexuality or gay life-style with others would more likely be open than secretive. Some people begin in secrecy, but such emotional tension builds that they feel they must tell someone or they'll explode under the pressure of their silence. The father of a young gay man with AIDS who had recently returned home after years of prostitution and drug use talked about his initial secrecy:

I didn't tell nobody for about three months. The only one I told was my supervisor on my job. Before that I had this pressure on me so bad [because] I couldn't talk to nobody.

For most family caregivers, the amount of secrecy or openness in going public changes over time. Caregivers who live more secretly in the beginning tend to move gradually toward a more assertive stance, and those who began openly usually become even more open. However, a few who live with secrecy never reveal themselves, such as one woman caring for her husband who concealed the information from everyone, even her family and children. Others live openly at first, but endure so much misery from stigma that they later withdraw into secrecy.

GOING PUBLIC FOR GAY CAREGIVERS

Since AIDS is associated with homosexuality, people often question the sexual orientation of AIDS caregivers. Gay caregivers in our study who weren't open about their sexuality were usually cautious about going public, especially outside of the gay community. A middle-aged teacher cared for his lover for a year before carefully disclosing the situation to someone at work:

There's only one person at work I have discussed this with— my boss. I had told him last summer that I was very stressed out—told him that the family was very sick, and so forth. He said, "Who?" which was actually more assertive, and I could have avoided that if I wanted to, but I decided to sort of go for it, and I said my lover's been very sick, and he all of a sudden started using the male pronoun. And so I just told him, and he's been pretty good about it.

Openly gay caregivers don't have to worry about concealing their sexuality. However, they do have to deal with the "guilt by association" phenomenon head-on, as this longtime lover of a man with AIDS, who describes himself as half of a "traditional yuppie gay couple," noted with frustration:

I could get upset with a lot of things people do. The fact that I am a partner with someone with AIDS, that they naturally assume that I am going to come down with AIDS, and that I too will die in the future, or the near future. They are looking at me like I'm this time bomb waiting to go off.

Parent caregivers of intravenous drug users and of gay children often consider themselves failures as parents, or are accused of poor parenting by others. Some of these parents feel guilty about their inability to prevent their child's homosexuality or drug use, and consequently their AIDS, as this mother noted:

He was the last person in the world we would ever expect to hear this from. The

first thing I did was to call a psychologist. There was so much guilt, and I wanted to learn more about the whys. The guilt was the heaviest load that I was carrying in the beginning [after learning he was gay]. The next questions were why, and who, and how did this happen?

Openness about the caregiving role or going public through community activity in AIDS work carries the additional risk of conflict between the person with AIDS and the caregiver. Sometimes a mismatch in ideas about privacy creates controversy in the relationship. For example, a caregiver might wish to become a voice for AIDS education in the community, to the dismay of the person with AIDS in her care who wants to keep colleagues at work from finding out he has the disease. When the caregiver and the person with AIDS agree and share strategies for controlling information, however, going public is usually accomplished without problems for the relationship. Yet some caregivers reluctantly comply with the sick person's preferences in order to keep the peace, as did one wife, a speech therapist:

He's stated many times that maybe the children would never have to know, so this is a secret. I've had to not give them any truth, and it's very difficult to live with all the lies. But he says that he can't handle [telling them the truth] right now and he couldn't handle losing them right now. For me, it would be easier if he had the ability to accept responsibility for it, and if telling people were not on my shoulders.

THE BENEFITS OF GOING PUBLIC

As the illness progresses and the person with AIDS needs more care, the benefits of being less secretive become more apparent. The caregivers in our study who went public suddenly found they had gained access to new resources. Now, a caregiver could ask AIDS volunteer services for help with errands or housekeeping. His or her tension, irritability, or fatigue at work could be explained, and a more flexible work schedule requested. And, he or she could get the comfort of emotional support from understanding people. A thirty-eight-year-old man told of his supervisor's pledge of support:

I went to work one morning, and I had this on my chest and I was crying. I told him, "I have to talk to you. What I have to tell you I haven't told nobody else. My son's got AIDS." And he sat across the table from me and he started crying. It shocked me. And he said, "If there is

anything I can do, let me know. I'm sorry, anything."

Acknowledgment from loved ones is another important personal benefit, as this young partner caregiver noted:

His parents have been real supportive. They came out to see us in May, and I had met them a couple of different times. They always address their letters to us, and they send me birthday letters. They are real supportive of me, and his mom has said several times that they were real glad that Tom and I were together, that Tom wasn't having to do all this by himself.

Assertive caregivers are sometimes rewarded with recognition and admiration from others for their caregiving accomplishments. Many caregivers take pride in the skills they develop as they provide care and successfully cope with the emotional challenge of caregiving. One middle-aged man, who was part of a local film about AIDS caregiving, felt satisfied with his nurturing abilities and proud of his advocacy skills:

I have developed certain strengths and abilities in different kinds of ways that are being called into play...and a number of people have said that Martin is very lucky that I have those. I'm real proud of myself.

SOCIAL RISKS AND BENEFITS

Our caregivers named several risks of remaining silent about their involvement with AIDS: inadequate health and social services, the perpetuation of homophobia and AIDS stigma, and the continued occurrence of AIDS. One young caregiver felt that speaking out about his caregiver role was a moral obligation, because silence would maintain the status quo:

> I really think that as long as AIDS remains a disease that "other people" deal with, then nothing changes, and we can continue to not provide people treatment and care, or education, or any of those kinds of things. Nothing will change until people say, "Oh, this affects me, or the guy I worked with, his lover had AIDS or somebody I went to school with."

Possible social benefits of openness the caregivers mentioned included better policies that govern AIDS care, and decreased homophobia and AIDS stigma because of greater public awareness of AIDS issues. Some caregivers have dedicated themselves to changing the cultural norms that keep sexual matters from open discussion, a silence which hinders AIDS prevention efforts. Several actively participate in ongoing educational projects about AIDS prevention, and in efforts to get rid of the fear and hostility surrounding AIDS.

Many feel the chief social benefit of openness is the creation of an AIDS community. Community identification gives caregivers a sense of belonging to a group with shared values and goals. A thirty-two-year-old gay lover told of his new-found sense of identity:

> I started really developing a community spirit. I was always [gay], but I was not outwardly gay, and I became a lot more involved with the gay community. Since then, I've devoted many hours of work, and now I call on the gay community. I see myself as part of the gay community now.

Shared values and goals influence the choices caregivers make when going public. For instance, caregivers in support groups often encourage each other to tell family and friends about their involvement with AIDS so they can get help with household tasks, gain emotional support, take care of their own needs, or make communication among family members a little more authentic. On the other hand, caregivers in political action groups are more likely to encourage openness in order to effect social change, such as raising public awareness of the difficulty for persons with AIDS in gaining access to experimental drugs.

However, not everyone we spoke to found his or her niche. The AIDS community in this study was not a single community, but instead was made up of overlapping yet diverse groups: the medical and health care, the biomedical research, the volunteer, and the gay communities. Consequently, community resources that appealed to one type of caregiver were often seen as uninviting to others.

For example, services delivered and used primarily by white gay men were often viewed as uncomfortable by heterosexual and parent caregivers, women, and people of color. As a result, many heterosexual caregivers, especially parents, said they felt extremely isolated without a sense of an AIDS community. A thirty-eight-year-old woman caring for a friend described the isolation and ambivalence a heterosexual AIDS caregiver often feels from straight people not involved with AIDS:

I feel a lot of distance from others. I'm a single, straight woman and live in the suburbs. You know, AIDS isn't something that my peer group—I'm the only one dealing with AIDS, and in a way, I'm bringing up something they don't want to deal with. And they do that by distancing from me. It's kind of hard. There's a part of me that wants to refuse to live the straight world of the city, and wants this suburb community to come into the [present].

In the best of circumstances, however, caregivers from diverse backgrounds joined together to create an AIDS community that transcended divisions of race, gender, and sexual preference. As caregivers, particularly female heterosexuals, sought services in the AIDS community, they often developed deep and lasting relationships with people in the gay community. One woman emphasized how much she cherished her friendships with gay men:

[As a straight woman] I have friendships that are based on AIDS. I have gay friends. My gay friends that I have formed based on AIDS are very special friendships.

For gay and lesbian caregivers in particular, the social benefit of openness is a heightened sense of community involvement. Many gay caregivers spoke of new-found pride in their sexual identity and membership in the gay community. A gay caregiver noticed a greater unity within the gay community as a result of AIDS:

All of the stuff that used to happen between gay men and lesbians and all of the political factionalism is not dropped away, but has lessened considerably.

These caregivers found community

identification necessary to spur activism and give themselves power to create social change. A twenty-three-year-old social worker caregiver described how he felt participating in his first AIDS march in Washington, DC:

The people with AIDS were first, and of course lovers, too. And so it was amazing for us to be at the head of this march, to see the incredible moving applause, and I still remember this one woman with tears in her eyes...it was just this sense of, "We're here and we have the support of this gigantic community." And even though we do not have the support of society yet, we have our community.

With enough education and understanding, the unreasonable terror of AIDS will abate, and persons with AIDS and the people who care for them will no longer experience fear and ridicule from others in our society. Until then, people involved with AIDS will continue to struggle with the negative consequences of going public. However, at the same time, people involved with AIDS will continue to benefit from the efforts of those who have broken the silence and worked for change.

THINGS TO THINK ABOUT

- Telling people that you are caring for a loved one with AIDS can bring strong reactions. Some people may avoid you or judge you, while others may offer help, kindness, and understanding.

- Don't take your friends' and family's first reaction as a permanent situation. With time, many people who care about you will come through.

- Remember that the most important reason to tell people is so others will understand what you're going through and offer support. Isolation can be an even heavier burden than other peoples' judgments.

- If you believe that your friends and family won't understand, consider counseling, support groups, and community groups such as Shanti, so that someplace in your life you can be honest about what you're going through.

- When you decide to tell others about your loved one with AIDS, consider how you will do it. If you stage information (select a certain amount and type of information and slowly paint a complete picture), it may help you gauge a person's response and prepare him or her for the impact of the real situation.

- Involvement in AIDS education and political activities can help you feel like you're making a difference. Public involvement in AIDS activities builds confidence, reduces feelings of helplessness, and makes changes that will improve the lives of all persons with AIDS and their caregivers. Skeptical or uninformed friends or co-workers, may become more tolerant when they see AIDS affects "real people" like you.

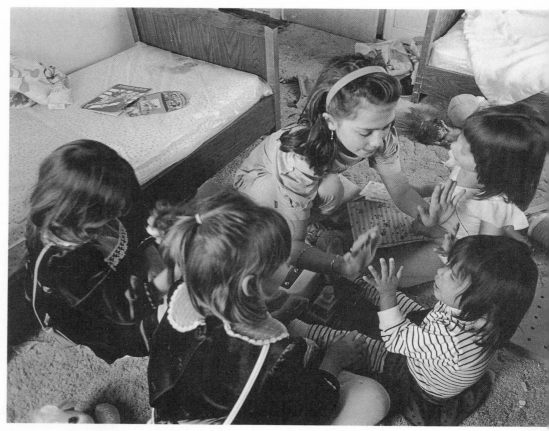

*Fear of getting or giving
the virus can cause
caregivers and people with
AIDS to overreact
and use unnecessary
precautions that have
nothing to do with how
the disease is transmitted.*

Containing the Spread of HIV

When people think of AIDS, they usually think of its communicability. AIDS is a contagious disease caused by Human Immunodeficiency Virus (HIV). HIV is transmitted from one person to another by contact with blood, semen, and vaginal fluids, or passed from an infected mother to an unborn child. The family caregiver's primary goal in containing the spread of HIV is to keep everyone free of the disease, or HIV negative: the caregiver, significant others, future offspring, other sexual partners of the person with AIDS, and the community at large. This chapter describes some of the methods caregivers use and some of the emotions they experience as they try to contain the spread of HIV.

WORKING THROUGH FEAR AND VULNERABILITY

At first, it is a sense of vulnerability to HIV infection that moves caregivers to contain the spread of HIV; as one wife caregiver in our study noted, "The fear of getting the disease was always there." Most caregivers work through fear and vulnerability by learning about the disease and how it is transmitted. Some caregivers, particularly people active in the gay community, already know a lot about AIDS when they begin caregiving. Other caregivers lack even the most basic knowledge about AIDS, and spend a great deal of energy searching for facts about the disease. Those who seek information often turn to health care providers, special caregiving classes, and AIDS community organizations.

Information alone helps some caregivers control their fear. As they learn more about AIDS, they realize that they can control its spread with certain behavioral changes and virtually eliminate their chances of contracting the disease.

For a few caregivers, however, facts don't allay anxiety. It's understandable that some people will feel threatened and terrified in the face of a deadly disease. Some caregivers need additional time, reassurance, and support to become comfortable with their closeness to AIDS, and to realize that the spread of HIV is something they can control.

DOING THINGS DIFFERENTLY

A caregiver learns to stop the spread of AIDS by doing everyday tasks differently. Disease-prevention techniques are incorporated into daily routine, and the early hypervigilant state becomes a calmer attentiveness and a sense of pride about controlling the fear. In most cases, these techniques eventually become habits, and caregivers perform them without even thinking about them. And, as caregivers become more confident in their ability to prevent the spread of HIV, their fear diminishes. Many methods caregivers use to contain the spread of HIV can be considered "correct" ways to prevent HIV transmission, based on scientific data. Parents of infants with AIDS use rubber gloves while changing the baby's diapers, instead of simply washing their hands afterwards. Caregivers use rubber gloves when contact with the sick person's body fluids is necessary— changing sheets soiled with diarrhea, or cleaning blood from an injection site. However, fear of getting or giving the virus can cause caregivers and people with AIDS to overreact and use unnecessary precautions that have nothing to do with how the disease is transmitted. For example, a caregiver might spend hours feverishly wiping household items with ammonia, or a person with AIDS may insist on completely separate food and utensils. Often caregivers will honor the sick person's requests even though they aren't consistent with current information about transmission:

We wash our own dishes by hand, and Don has decided that we have to use bleach—one cup of bleach to three cups of water. If you put your hand in there it will eat your nails off, and the fumes are so bad that you have to wash dishes with the windows wide open. He's got me doing the laundry. That's triple doing the laundry, because he takes his underwear and separates them so that all of his underwear is washed in another load. Why? I don't know. Underwear does not cross-infect.

Caregivers watch the sick person's behavior to make sure that he or she is acting safely, and try to encourage safe behavior in others. An ex-lover of a person with AIDS shared a house with him and another friend, and was afraid the sick person might not be cautious enough:

I had some fears about catching it, and I was really concerned that he wasn't using my razor and stuff like that, and the other day I even gave him my electric razor, but it was clear that he had used a blade. So I couldn't bring myself to ask him if he used a blade, and if he did use a blade, whose? Did he use his own? Instead, I had to play detective and go upstairs and make sure that the blade he used was not either Mike's or mine, which he didn't. I couldn't come right out and say, I just couldn't.

GETTING TESTED

As they work through their sense of vulnerability, many caregivers confront the possibility of their own HIV exposure. Caregivers who are sexual partners of persons with AIDS often feel fear and intense anger when they realize that they may have been unknowingly exposed to HIV by someone they trusted:

All of a sudden it became very real to me that I had been exposed for years, and how did I feel about that? That's when my anger really started.

The sick person's diagnosis raises the question of the HIV antibody status of others, particularly sexual partners and gay friends of a person with AIDS. Has the person with AIDS unknowingly infected his or her partner? A test for HIV isthe only way to answer this question:

I'm HIV negative, have been consistently, even though I shouldn't be. Dan and I had been together for four years

when he was diagnosed and he'd been completely healthy up to that point, so we had no reasons to practice protected sex. So I was exposed and I by all rights should have been infected, but I wasn't.

Most sexual partners and gay caregivers choose to be tested for HIV. Some may choose to be retested regularly, to reassure themselves that their preventative measures have worked. On the other hand, some caregivers hesitate to be tested. Their reluctance may have a variety of reasons, among them denial that they might be infected, the discomfort of facing their own mortality, or feeling overwhelmed by the person with AIDS's situation. One woman, a partner caregiver, spoke of the temptation to remain ignorant of her own HIV status:

I thought about not getting tested. Even though I'm going for anonymous testing, if I ever went to get health insurance and I lied about it and they found out, I'd never be insurable ever again.

Sometimes caregivers resist the test for HIV to protect the person with AIDS from the knowledge that he or she lives in a "two-positive home." The caregiver wants every bit of energy and attention focused on the person with AIDS, not on himself or herself. Also, a caregiver may want to spare the person with AIDS from guilt feelings about being the first to go, leaving the HIV-positive caregiver to deal with his or her illness alone. A middle-aged lover in the sixth year of his relationship with the person with AIDS told how he dealt with this problem:

> During the interview with the doctor, he asked me if I would have the test. And I told him no, and I told him why. He pressed and he pressed, and on my third visit of completing this physical, I finally said okay. I told him then that whatever the results are, I don't ever want Jim to know. I said that I don't want Jim to feel bad over the fact he has it and I don't, or I don't want him to feel bad thinking that I also have it and now we are a two-positive home.

RETHINKING SEX

For many caregivers, sex is the foremost issue of doing things differently. Even caregivers who aren't sexual partners of people with AIDS may start to think about the personal risks in their sexual behavior once they see the devastation of HIV infection. Choices about safer sex seem to depend on assessing the risk, and then settling on an acceptable level of personal risk. Caregivers who are sexual partners decide what steps should be taken toward safer sex,

keeping in mind the concerns of the person with AIDS:

> Sex is something that just happens once in a while now instead of on a regular schedule. I think he's afraid of infecting me, because one of the foremost things on his mind is that I stay negative.

Some caregivers we spoke to felt cheated or angry about the need to alter the sexual relationship. Others, such as this health care worker and long-time lover of a person with AIDS, met the new decisions with sadness and a sense of loss:

> The thing that has bothered me most is that on Don's part—it's his decision—he said, "Well, if we're not going to have sex, then I don't want the intimacy, either." Occasionally he wants a hug or a pat on the back, or [he'll] rub my leg, but there's not the closeness that there was before. It's there, but it's changed.

Most of the safer-sex strategies the caregivers in the study said they used were consistent with current public health recommendations. These public-health approved strategies include using condoms, avoiding anal or oral sex, practicing mutual masturbation, or abstaining from sex completely. Some said they augmented their new practices with sexual fantasy in order to become aroused. Some simply chose to find other (presumably HIV negative) sexual partners.

Since sexuality is an important part of life, it isn't surprising that major changes in sexual practice incur dramatic consequences. Some people have found that these changes actually benefit and enrich the sexual relationship. The relationship is refocused to include other forms of intimacy, adding new emotional dimension and placing less emphasis on the purely physical side of sexual activity:

Sex is less frequent, but it's better. We take more time at it. We take time to bring each other to arousal, more foreplay. We take more enjoyment out of it. It's not just a mechanical act any more. When we first got together, it was basically a lust relationship. Now we take emotional pleasure as well as physical pleasure in it. It's helped us keep the spark there.

On the other hand, some couples have found safer-sex changes difficult to handle. Sexual enjoyment and desire may suffer from the strict new rules:

There's hardly any spontaneity like there used to be. There is a lot more to think about: "This is what happens. These activities are off limits. This is risky for you, or this is risky for me," so the op-

tions are just not there any more. The options that are there seem so limited that it's really hard to change or make them spontaneous. I don't want to tell people about the limits, because I don't want people to not be having safe sex. But for us, it's just real strange. Since we had a closed relationship, it's changed a lot.

In open relationships, jealousy may consume the sick person whose caregiver seeks other sexual partners. Whatever the consequences of safer sex in a given relationship, it isn't surprising

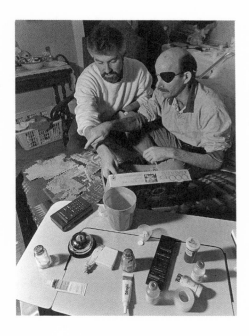

that behavioral change in such an emotional area can be difficult to sustain:

> *I don't particularly think it's romantic for me to become HIV positive and die with him. On the other hand, I do get carried away with my sexuality and don't always practice what I preach.*

Many caregivers are concerned about sexual transmission of HIV to others apart from themselves. Nonpartner caregivers try to encourage the people in their care to practice safer sex with their sexual partners. If the person with AIDS doesn't have one steady partner, the caregiver may try to persuade them not to have unsafe sex, as the person with AIDS may regret the decision not to protect his or her partner and suffer the guilt or anxiety of infecting others. From a broader perspective, some caregivers are ardently concerned about transmission to the community at large, and involve themselves in activities designed to educate the public about HIV transmission. One caregiver described himself as a "crusader for safe sex":

> *When Matt was first diagnosed, I went into a lot of community work. I worked the safe sex campaign in the gay bars. I mean, that was when a lot of unsafe sex was going on, and it was a reaction to what was going on for me.*

It's important to note that not all changes in sexual behavior are motivated by fear of HIV infection. Changes in the sexual relationship are often a result of the sick person's illness and the accompanying decreased sex drive:

> *We've almost stopped having sex. And there must be a couple of reasons for that. Initially Dan felt sick, and therefore didn't feel like having sex.*

Also, a caregiver may agree to do things differently to appease the person with AIDS, even if it's not a choice the caregiver would make:

> *Because we can't have sex regularly doesn't mean we can't touch each other. I know where it's coming from in him, and it's his paranoia and fear about the disease. I think he has some unreasonable fear that by some kind of intimacy he's going to contaminate me. I tested [HIV] positive anyway.*

It isn't easy to conquer the fear that accompanies the uncertainty of terminal illness. Fear is a natural reaction, and it takes considerable effort to loosen its powerful emotional hold. In most cases, with enough time, patience, and understanding, the fear of HIV infection evolves and diminishes, and the caregiver is able to focus on the more important aspects of caregiving:

I think I became more comfortable. It wasn't so predominant in my mind as time went on. So that, yes, by the time he was hospitalized I was sitting on his bed, and kissing him. This kind of thing. In the beginning, I don't know that I would have been that free to do those things. It was something I had to work into.

THINGS TO THINK ABOUT

- AIDS is a contagious disease. It's normal to feel afraid and confused about protecting yourself and others, particularly when you first start taking care of your loved one. As you learn more and gain experience, you will become more comfortable knowing what to do.

- Facts alone may not be enough to change strong initial reactions to the contagiousness of AIDS. Learn about precautions and use them faithfully, and try to balance your fear of contagion with trust that these precautions really do work.

- If you're in a sexual relationship with a loved one with AIDS, this relationship may become strained as you or your partner worry about your becoming infected. Talk to each other about these fears. Be cre-

ative, find new ways to express love, and realize you can still have an intimate relationship with someone who is HIV positive.

- If you've engaged in high-risk behavior, you may want to consider getting tested for HIV. Knowing you are negative can free you from unnecessary worry and let you be more comfortable in your caregiving role. If you find you are positive, early diagnosis can alter the decisions you make about your health care.

- If you choose to be tested, anonymous testing and counseling is available through the local public health department. You can also ask your private health care provider about testing.

- You may find yourself monitoring your loved one's AIDS prevention behavior. Make sure both of you know the facts, and give the person with AIDS a chance to talk about any difficulty he or she has with safe practices. Be honest about your concerns, but remember that criticism and negative judgement will usually lead to conflict between the two of you.

AIDS Facts

1. AIDS stands for Acquired Immune Deficiency Syndrome, a condition caused by the Human Immunodeficiency Virus, or HIV.

2. AIDS destroys the body's natural defenses against infection and disease.

3. AIDS can affect anybody, regardless of age, race, sex, or sexual preference.

4. The HIV virus dies quickly outside the body. It is easily killed with soap and water and common disinfectants.

5. While using a latex condom during sexual intercourse can help reduce the possibility of contracting HIV, condoms aren't foolproof.

6. Only a qualified health professional can diagnose AIDS.

AIDS IS SPREAD BY:

- sharing intravenous needles or syringes with an infected person, or getting stuck accidentally with a needle carrying contaminated blood
- having sexual intercourse with an infected person
- an infected mother transmitting it to her baby during pregnancy, birth, or breastfeeding
- receiving contaminated blood, blood products, or transplanted organs (although this possibility is very rare, since blood donations are screened, it still occurs)

AIDS IS NOT SPREAD BY:

- Coughing or sneezing
- Hugging or casual skin contact
- Using toilet seats, doorknobs, or swimming pools
- Shaking hands
- Sharing food or utensils
- Contact with animals or insects (including mosquitoes)
- Donating blood

References

Eidson, Ted (Ed.) *The AIDS Caregiver's Handbook*. St. Martin's Press, New York, 1988.

Monette, Paul. *Borrowed Time: An AIDS Memoir*. Avon Books, New York, 1988.

Felder, Leonard. *When a Loved One Is Ill: How To Take Better Care of Your Loved One, Your Family, and Yourself*. NAL Books, New York, 1990.

Moffatt, Bettyclare. *When Someone You Love Has AIDS*. NAL Penguin Inc., New York, 1986.

Sommers, Tish, and Laurie Shields. *Women Take Care: The Consequences of Caregiving In Today's Society*. Triad Publishing Co., Gainesville, Florida, 1987.

Need Help or Information about AIDS?
Call the National AIDS Clearinghouse: 1-800-458-5231
They provide AIDS general information, business and workplace information, AIDS services and educational resources information, AIDS clinical trial information, and information about how to order AIDS publications.

About the Study

We talked to people who represented just about every possible relationship with the person with AIDS. Many were caring for a spouse, life partner or lover; these couples included both heterosexual and gay relationships.

We also talked to parents of young children with AIDS, as well as parents now caring for grown children who found themselves ill and alone, and sought the refuge of their original families. In this group, parents and siblings, particularly mothers and sisters, took on the caregiver role.

Plus, we saw something we believe is unique to AIDS: a large representation of friends who took on this challenging role, which in our culture is usually left to spouses, partners, or biological family.

About one-third of the caregivers in our study were partners in gay relationships, and a little under half were friends or former lovers; the rest were the parents, spouses, heterosexual life partners, brothers or sisters, or other biological family members of the person with AIDS. Most of the caregivers lived in the same household with the person with AIDS, and most of these households included other people, such as the caregiver's partner, child, or housemates.

The group of people interviewed reflects the demographics of AIDS in the Seattle area. Two-thirds were men and one-third were women. Most were white. Approximately 50% of the caregivers were employed full-time, and 20% part-time outside the home, with incomes ranging from under $10,000 to over $40,000.

The caregivers ranged in age from 22 to 65. Approximately 50% were under the age of 36. Fifty-seven percent had less than a college degree.

Throughout the entire study, all caregivers' identities were kept confidential.

After the findings were analyzed, we asked a number of people to evaluate whether we had portrayed accurately what life is like for family caregivers of persons with AIDS. Caregivers who had participated in the study, caregivers who hadn't participated in the study, and professionals and volunteers working with AIDS and family caregiving helped us review and critique the validity of our descriptions.